ALONG WITH A BALANCED DIET AND EXERCISE

DANCE a little longer,

LAUGH a little louder,

HOLD HANDS a little tighter,

KISS like your heart wants to thunder,
and find the

HAPPINESS that thrills you with wonder.

Elahe Toosi & Lowell Campbell

ALONG WITH A BALANCED DIET AND EXERCISE

Our take on a healthy lifestyle

Elahe Toosi, MSc &
Lowell Campbell, PhD

La Costa, California

Ameh IP

Ameh IP books may be purchased for educational, business, or sales promotional use. Special discounts are available on bulk purchases by corporations, associations, and others. For details, please contact the publisher at Ameh IP, P.O. Box 131654, La Costa, CA 92013.

FIRST EDITION

Designed by Elahe Toosi and Lowell Campbell.

Title: Along with a balanced diet and exercise: Our take on a healthy lifestyle / Elahe Toosi, MSc & Lowell Campbell, PhD.

Description: First edition. | La Costa, CA: Ameh IP, Published 2023. | Printed in the United States of America.

Identifiers: Library of Congress Control Number: 2023933054 | ISBN 979-8-9877600-0-0 (hardcover) | ISBN 979-8-9877600-1-7 (paperback) | ISBN 979-8-9877600-2-4 (eBook)

Subject: Healthy Lifestyle. | Health/Weight Loss. | Metabolism/Energy. | Correct Food.

Contents

FOREWORD

Elahe (Ellie) and I (Lowell) felt compelled to write this book to answer the numerous inquiries about our lifestyle. We have reached a point where it is more practical to produce a synopsis of our answers to these queries, and thereby provide a more complete and general response. A comprehensive elucidation has proved to be too big a project, so our first book of what could be a series will focus on health and diet. This choice is fitting, since our most frequently received inquiries are directed to how Ellie maintains her stunning figure. To this end, we outline some basic principles, explain why most diet plans are doomed to fail, and provide our way in substantial detail.

PREFACE

When you see television advertisements about diets and diet aids, they nearly always include a line such as "Our diet product blah blah blah ... along with a balanced diet and exercise". Consider the possibility that you might get the same result by just having a balanced diet and exercise.

ACKNOWLEDGEMENTS

I (Lowell) wish to thank Elahe for 20 wonderful years, and a life and future together forever. And I (Elahe) am grateful to Lowell for all those wonderful years of showing me what love is, and I too wish a life and future together forever.

Chapter 1: Introduction

The frequent curiosity about our lives has come as a surprise to us. We always went about our business quietly and unobtrusively, but over time started to notice unusual attention from others. At first, I thought I was just being paranoid. I started noticing people that seemed to be following us around in supermarkets. Surely, they were only coincidently shopping around the same aisles. But one time a woman followed us so long and bought so many of the things we did, that I finally turned to Ellie lifted my arms and said: "Did you see that?". It turned out Ellie has been noticing it as much as I had.

This attention continued in other forms. People we did not know would honk and wave when they saw us kiss at stoplights. Walking together by the beach, a man we had never met came up to us and said: "You are so lucky. You look like the King and Queen out for a walk". Another time in a completely different town we were just visiting, another man saw us and said: "You look important. If importance had a look, it would be you". Two women came up to Ellie and said: "We see you around town. You give us hope". Another woman told us: "I love how close you two are. I am going to go home and hug my husband". People we did not know would ask about details of our lives that they had heard about from others. But why were they so curious? Nothing we did seemed that unusual. We held hands when we walked. We would hug each other while shopping, and kiss occasionally. Nothing unusual it seemed, but apparently it is. When we started looking around, we saw it was unusual. We rarely saw couples shopping, and when they were, they barely paid attention to each other. What was ordinary to us was not ordinary to most other people. Happiness seems to be a rare commodity.

More and more people would ask us for advice, or say how we were such an adorable couple, merely because we seemed so happy together. They usually assumed we were newly married, on a honeymoon, an anniversary, or had just been drinking a lot. They were further surprised to learn we were always like this. It was no public show or special occasion, that is just how we are. But the sad part is why should a happy couple be so unusual? Happiness should be such an ordinary thing that it should not stand out. Why aren't most people happy, and how can we help others be happy?

Written recorded history goes back about five thousand years, but modern humans have existed largely unchanged with the same level of intelligence for over a hundred thousand years. Thus, we have a hundred thousand years of tradition and oral history originating from knowledge accumulated throughout that time. People of the current era often like to pretend that because we are surrounded by technological gadgets that we are somehow smarter and cope better in our human interactions. In truth, we only have a wealthier lifestyle not a better one. So, here we do not claim ultimate ontological truth, or to not repeat things others may have long said, but our unique take on life may benefit some people.

This book details practical and philosophical principles that have worked for us. We do not claim a miracle cure; we only outline ideas and aspirational ideals that have worked for us for 20 years. Looking at every aspect of lifestyle proved to be too big a subject for one book, so we decided to limit the scope of this book to health. This book is targeted to individuals who wish to make a long-term effective change to their lifestyle for the benefit of improved overall health and/or weight loss.

Our philosophy is to eat what you like, but the highest quality version of it, and not too much. In our Lowellie™ Way for a healthy lifestyle, we recommend reducing fat savers and increasing fat burners. The Lowellie™ Way is focused on choosing the correct food within the Calories required for your ideal weight while creating a more energetic you. Correct food is good for you and tastes good. We recommend you eat correct food to produce premium food fuel in your body for generating optimal burnable energy, i.e., adenosine triphosphate (ATP) for performing your daily activities.

Many people do not know about the effects of the food they eat on their metabolism, so they often choose foods pushed through the media. As such, the journey to weight loss for many can be a struggle. Our way is simple, knowledge, so you trust your own judgment not "Experts".

We explain the philosophical underpinnings of our way based on how the human body has been optimized to live in a preindustrial natural environment over millions of years. We explain why this biological predisposition dooms most diets to failure. We make recommendations on how to succeed in maintaining a balanced diet of correct food in a correct amount for a long-term healthy and happy lifestyle. No need for short-term weight loss programs and useless dietary supplements or diet products. However, some foods vitamins and minerals in moderation may need to be included in your diet, as your body may not synthesize them in the quantities required to maintain proper metabolism.

Your success often comes down to how much to eat, what to eat, and better yet what not to eat. We will outline our way, the Lowellie™ Way. We further outline how we spend a typical day and provide some philosophical underpinnings for our lifestyle. Our goal is to create a short handbook like Strunk and White, a famous writing handbook, but for a healthy diet.

Chapter 2: 20 Years

Love, dance, and correct food. Lucky us—we must have done something good in our childhoods, or maybe it is what we eat ☺.

Ellie was told "It's not possible.", when she informed a friend that we had been together and happily so and as close as we are for 20 years. She thought we had just met and were retired and not working, but quite to the contrary, we work hard all day every day and spend all the time together. So, what is it that makes our lives so wonderful? Well for us it is being together all the time and enjoying the time together. We work together, eat, exercise, shop, go to dentists and doctors together, recreate, and rest together all day every day.

On a typical day we have our breakfast and go off to work. Our breakfast generally comprises a combination of correct foods such as egg whites, whole eggs, spinach, ham, turkey, smoked salmon, whey protein powder, chocolate covered strawberries, and dried plums. We work together at our own business, so we spend the morning doing our tasks for the day, then head home for lunch.

We work together at our own business because freedom is priceless. As you would expect, working together is hard. You cannot fire your spouse; however, you do not have a close relationship by avoiding hard things. If you pretend to never disagree, you have a pretend relationship. A strong relationship is not built on magic, but rather on reality. That is not to say that it must always be difficult. A friend of ours once said "You have to work at a relationship.", and some other books have even proposed relationship performance reviews. No, it is really not work and does not require planning or special effort if your spouse is the focus of your life. You do not need to consult a performance review checklist to figure out what your spouse wants if you are close. If you run your relationship like a business, your spouse is probably going to look for a better deal.

For lunch we usually make salads and meat dishes with correct foods such as fish, turkey, avocado, beats, spinach, lettuce, brussels sprouts, asparagus, almonds, pistachios, and walnuts. Also, fruits such as apples, pears, persimmons, and grapes. Then we take a short afternoon nap. Napping even for a few minutes could improve your health because it can decrease your stress levels and your blood pressure, improve your ability to remember things, improve alertness, and can kick your caffeine boost up a notch too. Napping has been part of human culture from the beginning but has been neglected in our modern society. Romans and Greeks took a nap each day just after lunch. In many countries around the world people still do take a nap after lunch, some close their shops for a short nap.

In the afternoon, we usually work from home until exercise time in the early evening. We workout 4 days a week and dance tango at least twice a week. You must take care of your health, and exercise daily. At the time of writing this book many women used to go to yoga classes and hug the yoga mats they bring like they were babies in their arms, but yoga mats do not hug back. At the gym, each time we met when either of us was running around the track, we kissed because we missed each other so much. We dance tango by the beach in view of a pier with lights like the Starry Night Over the Rhone painting of nighttime Arles by Vincent van Gogh.

After exercise or dancing, we have dinner and relax and watch TV to prepare to sleep. For dinner we mostly make soups, salads, and meat dishes from variety of correct foods such as chicken, ham, lettuce, cabbage, carrots, onion, garlic, blue cheese, eggs, and avocado;

plus, desserts: apples, pears, persimmons, berries, grapes, yogurt, and milk. Occasionally we have flex foods: steak, ground beef burger, chili, spaghetti, pizza, cioppino, or Persian food. We mostly make them at home with the basic ingredients chosen from correct foods when possible. So, we can have our not-so-correct food and eat it too.

Strangely, everywhere we go we draw attention, even though we try hard to be invisible. We do what we do for ourselves, and not for show, but people seem to have to pay attention to love. It is truly something to have a romance that is better than any story, movie, or song you have ever imagined, read about, or heard. When we say 20 years, they cannot believe it. They say things like: "You look good, we want to eat what you eat", "We want to dance like you dance", and "We want to kiss like you kiss". When we hear that, it makes us motivated to write more because people mostly do understand what they need to do to be happy. They just need to hear or read more about it.

Chapter 3: Trust Yourself not "Experts"

There have been numerous diet fads that have been recommended by "Experts" throughout the ages. Some notorious ones include soda pop, which was a patent medicine with added soda water, and breakfast cereal that was invented as a digestive aid. Now they are both mostly sugary candy food. Even assuming they have good motives, we should not assume they are always right or that their recommendations have the same effect on everyone or even most people. There is no guarantee their recommendations apply to our individual circumstances.

Scientists make many assumptions when performing food studies. For example, they may test for one variable or one chemical and assume their design-of-experiments can eliminate all other variables. For example, they may set the amount of a particular food or chemical eaten and try to randomize all other factors. This may not be possible in the real world. They may also conflate causation and correlation, which is assuming two events happening in sequence or combination means one must cause the other, which should not be automatically assumed. For example, there have been studies in the past that showed drinking sugary soda pop correlated to the test subjects losing weight. The argument was that the test subjects would eat fewer Calories overall if they drank sugary soda, but do you really believe that? There are thousands, millions and perhaps even billions of different chemicals operating within our bodies that interact in ways that are generally impossible to accurately model and may be impossible to approximate. Furthermore, psychological response and feedback add even more complexity. The difficulty of making an accurate analysis is generally downplayed, so you should listen to any "Expert" opinion with skepticism.

Fad dieting requires concentration to resist what your body is demanding or requiring. Your higher brain functions allow humans to forgo immediate needs for longer term gains, but you need to understand what your body is demanding or requiring, or your body will find a way to make you give it what it wants. The human body has been optimized to live in a preindustrial natural environment full of hardships and dangers over millions of years. This biological predisposition dooms most fad diets to failure because they focus on quick results that do not conform to your body's long-term needs. For a weight loss diet to work, your body should be made to feel safe for an extended time to be willing to reduce reserves such as fat. As such, any change in lifestyle should be over an extended time to allow adjustment time. In the long run, your body including your conscious and subconscious mind will tell you or make you conform to what it wants. You are the only one who has access to the feedback from your body, and that feedback will probably be the best information you can get. So, that is why you need to trust your own judgment not "Experts". We will give you tools to help you do so—knowledge.

The title of our book refers to the endless number of advertisements that say, "use our blah-blah diet supplement or diet products" "along with a balanced diet and exercise". If you have a balanced diet and exercise, you will get good results regardless of the product they foist on you. So, we skip the fad diets and just go straight to a balanced diet and exercise.

Most of us know people who can eat ice cream, cake, and whatever else they want and still not gain weight. At the other extreme are people who seem to gain weight no matter how little they eat. Why? What allows one person to remain thin without effort but demands that another struggle to avoid gaining weight or regaining the pounds he or she has lost previously? On a simple level, your weight depends on the number of Calories you consume, how many of those Calories you store, and how many you burn up. But each of these factors is influenced by a combination of genes and environment. Both can affect your physiology (such as how fast you burn Calories) as well as your behavior (the types of foods you choose to eat, for instance). The interplay between all these factors begins at conception and continues throughout your life. That interplay is specific to you, so to be effective, your lifestyle should be customized by you based on knowledge of how your body works not just based on a generic template from "Experts".

As we previously explained, we want you to eat the correct food to provide premium fuel to the cells in your body for generating optimal burnable energy, i.e., ATP for performing your daily activities. Most people do not know about the effects of the food they eat on their metabolism, so they often choose whatever food that some in the diet industry try to sell them. As such, the journey to weight loss for most is a struggle. Our way is simple, knowledge, so you trust your own judgment not "Experts". Because you are the best expert on you.

In the rest of this book, we will outline what our way, the Lowellie™ Way is, why it works, and give a limited exploration of related metabolic biochemistry in the context of metabolism as a foundational basis. Metabolic biochemistry is the chemical process that converts the food you eat such as protein, fat, and carbohydrate (carbs) to burnable energy within your cells to maintain your life. Metabolism is the sum of the types of metabolic biochemistry reactions in your body. The knowledge of metabolism never fails to amaze us. You too will find many aha moments when you discover it. Most importantly, with the knowledge of what is in what you eat and how it can affect your metabolism, you will most likely be encouraged to choose the correct foods as we will explain later. Correct foods and activities are "a balanced diet and exercise" that maintains a long-term healthy and happy lifestyle with lots of burnable energy.

Chapter 4: The "Magic" of Achieving a Healthy Weight

In modern times our abundant food, technological entertainment, conveniences, and sedentary lifestyles lead most people to be above their ideal weight often to an unhealthy degree. Eating robot drone delivered pizza and soda while playing virtual reality video games can pack on the pounds. In counterpoise to that, you need to be careful about your health, so you live a long and active life. There are many components to staying healthy, but here we will focus on food and weight, and how you develop a preference for quality of food that helps you, over quantity that may hurt you.

Most of us are not at our ideal weight or have difficulty maintaining it. People tend to select their chosen weight based more on fashion than on what is ideal for health. The most fashionable weight often depends on what indicates that you are healthy or wealthy. Showing you having lots to eat in the form of fat could indicate health and wealth as it has throughout most of history, but so can being thin, which may show you have a wealth of leisure time to exercise and take care of your health. The fashion of weight has changed many times through history. You should want to keep an ideal weight based on health because it makes your body function better, not necessarily because of fashion. You can usually cover fashion requirements with clothes. An ideal weight for your body can be defined as a weight that makes your body function best.

Good health is the magic. You can make the magic by simply keeping your Calories within the Calories required for your ideal weight as opposed to making radical changes in your diet as some advocate. For most of us that means decreasing total Calories over a length of time by methods we will outline in this chapter. Strategic choices in what foods you eat to get those Calories and other nutrients can make this an enjoyable experience.

For practical purposes, to reach your ideal weight over time, you may choose an intermediate target weight different than or the same as your ideal weight. For example, your ideal weight and target weight may be the same if you are overweight by a little, so in this book we may use target weight and ideal weight interchangeably. However, if you are overweight by a lot, you may choose a target weight higher than your ideal weight as an intermediate step to get to your ideal weight.

For example, an ideal weight for a 5' 6" (1.68 m) female may range from 117 to 143 pounds (53-65 kilograms). You can determine what your ideal weight should be by consulting Appendix A of this book or similar weight charts readily available on the Internet. Internet weight charts are not always based on the same concepts, so they are not all identical but are usually reasonably similar. Weight charts are generally based on age, sex, and height, and you can choose an ideal weight based on your own philosophy as to how much of your total body weight (fat + everything else) should be fat.

Fat includes necessary body fat and reserve body fat. Necessary body fat is needed to protect the body from diseases and physically protect organs from bruising damage. Reserve body fat is an additional fat that presents no risk to health but rather provides a store of fuel for the body to use when needed. Everyone needs some reserve fat for non-ordinary activity such as extended exertion, emotional aggravation, and illness. Body fat significantly more than the necessary and reserve body fat can lead to serious health problems such as heart disease and diabetes.

Bear in mind, body fat is stored in your body when you consume more Calories than you use from all foods you eat not just from dietary fat. It is up to you to keep your Calories in check to maintain an optimal level of body fat for your health. While there may be no official standard for acceptable body fat percentage values, a range of 10 to 20 percent for men and 18 to 28 percent for women may be good ranges to set goals around. You can use body fat calculators available on the Internet to calculate your body fat percentage.

Many people cannot lose weight because they either do not know why they gain weight in the first place, or they know it is because they eat too much but cannot stop. In either case they cannot lose weight because they eat more than they need, thus the excess food gets stored in the form of fat. Many people eat impulsively because they are not happy with something in their lives and use excessive food as a short-term comfort at the expense of potential long-term damage. Even being moderately above your ideal weight increases wear on your joints and causes your heart to pump extra blood, increasing the load on your heart. Some people resort to short-term weight loss programs that may work while they focus on the program, but then they gain back what they lost because they cannot maintain that level of concentration over the long-term. Really, no one can maintain such a level of concentration long-term. Just think of all the famous athletes and celebrities who fall apart after they passed their peak.

Healthy living must be an enjoyable part of life. To be successful, you should know what you need to do and why. You should know the fundamental mechanism of how your body works and why what you eat matters. Losing weight should always be through a change in lifestyle not just a diet. You should permanently change what you eat, rather than temporarily reduce how much you eat to lose weight.

Since human bodies evolved to handle the variability and scarcity of food in the natural world, your body sees a quick reduction in food as starvation and will therefore try to regain back that weight and more to protect you from the next famine. By very slowly and steadily changing your food intake to match the steady state amount required to maintain your target weight, your body will recognize that you are living in a benign environment, and not require you to store extra fat. If possible, you should plan to lose weight over a period of years rather than a few weeks or months. Afterall, you did not gain that weight in a few weeks or months in the first place.

Many people on quick-fix diets go on a "yo-yo" dieting spree, which is a pattern of rapidly losing and then regaining weight, and most importantly getting discouraged from repeatedly failing to keep it off. They may even get into a long-term struggle with weight and a greater risk of obesity. This is because during the evolutionary process, humans developed a way of long-term survival. We evolved mechanisms to reserve fat for rainy days and not to reduce fat reserves unless the environment is safe for doing so. Short-term weight loss will almost inevitably be regained just as quickly.

In contrast, *Lowellie*™ Way offers a long-term weight loss plan where you most likely enjoy the process, enjoy your food, and enjoy the resulting happiness, so you will stay motivated to keep the magic.

4.1 *Lowellie*™ Way: A recipe for success

Even if a particular diet works for one person it may not work for another. The human body is rather like a highly sophisticated machine. It operates to maintain the well-being of a specific individual based on a set of specific parameters that make up that individual. The Lowellie™ Way in essence is a structured method of replacing larger Calorie quantities of lower quality food with lower Calorie quantities of higher quality food. To wit:

Eliminate bread! We want you to be successful in losing weight right out of the gate. To start with, the most important factor in our way is to eliminate bread and reduce other carbs from your daily diet. No matter how much you love bread, you probably can put it on hold for a little while until you can fit into your "skinny clothes" again. The good news is that it does not take long before you can fit in your skinny clothes, and better yet reward yourself with a big loaf of bread!! Just kidding, a moderate slice—remember, live a steady lifestyle.

Find out how many excess Calories you eat per day: While cutting down on bread and other carbs, it is important to realize how many excess Calories you eat per day. Some people do not even know how much they overeat, but they do know they are overweight. The trick is now to cut the extra Calories, and the question is by how much? Most people do not know how many more Calories they eat compared to what their body needs. They keep saying: "I eat healthy, but why do I gain weight?". As a basic principle, losing weight means simply less Calories coming into your body than going out. You can follow these six simple steps to find out how many more Calories you are eating than your body needs: 1) list each food item you eat in one day, 2) list the Calories for each food item, 3) calculate your total Calorie intake per day from the list in step 2, 4) find your ideal weight from Appendix A: Ideal Weight Chart or similar charts, 5) use a Calorie calculator from the Internet to find out how many Calories you need to maintain your ideal weight in one day, and finally 6) subtract your total Calorie intake per day you calculated in step 3 from the Calories you need to maintain your ideal weight in one day that you calculated in step 5. The result is likely a number that may surprise you with how many more excess Calories you eat than your body needs.

Reduce your daily Calories: Now that you know how many excess Calories you eat, it is time to reduce it. The safest way to handle a Caloric reduction for fat loss is to reduce your intake by a small quantity and then be consistent. To lose weight safely, you need to consume less than your daily Caloric needs for your current weight but not less than your Basal Metabolic Rate (BMR). BMR represents the minimal Calorie number you need for involuntary body functions when at rest, and it is the equivalent of figuring out how much gas an idle car consumes while parked. The daily Caloric needs include the BMR plus what you need for daily activity. That is your starting point. However, as you lose weight, your BMR will change accordingly. As such, it will likely be necessary to adjust your Calorie intake plan to continue making progress. You can use calculators readily available on the Internet to estimate both your daily Caloric needs and your BMR.

Generally, if you are a person within an average range for height, and age you may be able to reduce your Caloric intake by about 200-600 Calories until you reach your ideal weight. To put this in an interesting context, the Calorie content of a doughnut is about 450 which is close to that of a stick of dynamite. The difference is that the energy from the dynamite is released instantly when ignited, while the doughnut releases its energy content in the body more slowly. So, you don't blow up from a doughnut, at least not instantly or literally. Suppose your current weight is 170 pounds (77 kilograms) and your BMR is 1700 Calories. Assuming a moderate physical activity level, suppose the requirement in a day for your body to stay the same is 2500 Calories. Now assume your ideal weight is 150 pounds (68 kilograms), and you want to lose 20 pounds (9 kilograms) to reach it. You could safely reduce your daily Calorie intake by 500 Calories which keeps your Calorie consumption per day above your BMR. Each pound (0.45 kilogram) of your weight is equal to about 3500 Calories and there are 70,000 Calories in 20 pounds (9 kilograms). So, if your net Calories per day are -500 Calories, you will lose 3500 Calories in 7 days, which is about one pound (0.45 kilogram) per week or 1/8 gallon (1 pint, 0.5 liters) of volume in 2 weeks. And you will lose 20 pounds (9 kilograms) or 2.5 gallons (10 liters) of volume in 140 days or less than 5 months. Not too bad. You may choose your net Calories to be any amount you can manage. If you choose to reduce 200 Calories a day, you will lose 20 pounds (9 kilograms) in 350 days or about a year - not too bad either. The point is to change the direction of your weight toward slow-steady reduction. Weight reduction is not a race, it is a lifestyle!

For another example, measure your weight (e.g., 136 pounds/62 kilograms), find out how many Calories you need per day to maintain that weight (e.g., 2100 Calories). Find your ideal weight (e.g.,130 pounds/59 kilograms). Subtract your current weight from your ideal weight to find out how much weight you need to lose (e.g., 6 pounds/3 kilograms). Choose a target weight that you think you can live with. In this case you may choose the target weight to be equal to the ideal weight since your current weight and the ideal weight are only 6 pounds (3 kilograms) apart. Reduce your Calories intake until you reach your ideal weight. If you need to lose 6 pounds (3 kilograms) you need to lose 21,000 Calories. If your net Calories are -300/day, you will reach your target weigh in 70 days. Then measure your weight at least every week to keep track of your progress. To maintain your ideal weight (e.g., 130 pounds/59 kilograms), your daily Calorie intake should be 1,800, which is the 2,100 Calories you needed to maintain your original weight minus 300 Calories.

If you are significantly overweight, your target weight and your ideal weight may be different. You can make your target weight a moving target until you reach your ideal weight, so you do not lose too much weight too soon. For example, if you are a 5' 4" (163 cm) woman and weighs 320 pounds (145 kilograms) you need about 4,200 Calories per day to maintain your weight. Your ideal weight is between 108-132 pounds (49-60 kilograms). If you choose the higher end of your ideal weight, 132 pounds (60 kilograms), then you would need about 2,200 Calories per day to maintain your ideal weight.

But you have a challenging task of losing about 188 pounds (85 kilograms) to get to the 132 pounds. To make the task doable, you can choose a target weight that is way more than the ideal weight. You can target 280 pounds (127 kilograms) which is 150 pounds (68 kilograms) more than your ideal weight. In this example, to begin with, you will be targeting to lose about 40 pounds (18 kilograms) instead of targeting the whole 188 pounds (85 kilograms). 40 pounds (18 kilograms) is still a lot of weight to lose. To put it in perspective, 8 pounds (4 kilograms) means losing 1 gallon (4 liters) of volume around your body. Being 40 pounds (10 kilograms) overweight is like having 5 gallons (20 liters) of milk tied around your waist!

You can lose the first 40 pounds (18 kilograms) or about 140,000 Calories in about 280 days by cutting 500 Calories a day and move the target for the next 40 pounds (or whatever amount you choose) until you get to or near your ideal weight. This way you can make the target reachable, so you can have some success, but not so easy that achieving it does not feel like an accomplishment.

As you move to the next target weight you can cut your daily Calories based on each target weight but keep it simple for purpose of clarity. For example, you may cut your Calories by about 500 Calories a day, then you can lose all the 188 pounds (85 kilograms,) or about 658,000 Calories in about 3.5 years or less. Bear in mind that you weigh about 50 pounds (23 kilograms) less each year while you are working toward your ideal weight.

By cutting 500 Calories at each new target weight, you could reduce your daily Calorie intake while staying above your BMR ranging from 2,200 Calories at 320 pounds (145 kilograms) to 1,400 Calories at 132 pounds (60 kilograms). To maintain your ideal weight at 132 pounds (60 kilograms), you need to maintain 2,200 Calories daily which is 2,000 Calories less than what you needed to maintain your original weight at 320 pounds (145 kilograms). 2,000 Calories less is not only a lot healthier for you but is also more economical from money saved on food!

Make a tool to manage your Calorie intake: To reach your ideal weight successfully, it is not only important to know how to reduce your daily Calories, but it is also important to be able to do it easily. Many people jump off the weight loss bandwagon before they reach the destination because they do not have an easy-to-use tool to effectively keep track of their Calories. To that end, you need an easy-to-use Calorie management tool to keep track of your Calorie intake easily, because you may only be as effective as your tools.

A Quick Calorie Chart (QCC) listing Calories for foods we eat has proven to be a helpful tool for us. An example of our QCC is listed in Appendix B. You can make your own QCC tool so you can quickly determine how much of everything you are eating each day and how much you can eat to achieve or to maintain the weight you want whether it is your ideal weight or your target weight.

To keep it simple, list Calories in your QCC per unit of food item or per unit of measurement that is easy for you to remember, so you can easily visually estimate the Calories in your food portion. Did you know there are 7 Calories in each almond? 130 Calories in one slice of toasted bread? 2.5 Calories in each green bean? But the good news is that you need to measure the Calories only for a short while because you will quickly learn how many Calories each food item has and how much is too much. For example, list the Calories in one almond, and in one oz of fish.

Substitute your food items with correct food: As we will discuss in Chapter 12, you can continue eating the same food you have been eating, only the correct version of it, within the Calories of your ideal weight. Once you make your QCC from the food items you like, you can update it by substituting your food items with better quality food. For example, if you like them, you can substitute: some nuts for bread, almond butter for peanut butter, avocado for mayonnaise, fresh fruit for fruit juice, or fresh olive oil or avocado oil (fruit oils) for vegetable oils. Over time, populate your QCC with correct food as you learn more about them.

Have a proper amount of each macronutrient: It is also important to have a proper amount of each macronutrient according to your daily needs. Macronutrients generally comprise carbohydrates, fats, and proteins. Assemble each of your meals out of correct types and amounts of protein, fat, and carbs. According to some research literature, the recommended dietary reference intake (DRI) for nutrition is 10-35% from protein, 20-35% from fats, and 45-65% from carbs based on your daily caloric need.

For example, if your ideal weight is 175 pounds (80 kilograms) and your daily Caloric intake is about 2,275.

You may need about 63-200 grams of protein, about 50-88 grams of fat, and about 255-284 grams of carbs daily. However, the intake of food should be based on your objective, whether you want to improve your general health, to lose weight, or gain muscle. For example, if you plan to lose weight, your carbs intake should be lower than the DRI that may be about 50-150 grams a day. If you plan to make more muscles, you may choose a high end of the protein intake range. You can determine a range for your daily macronutrient needs by using calculators readily available on the Internet, which is a good starting point. However, if you want to calculate a more specific amount of each macronutrient customized to your daily needs, we show you more ways in Chapter 10.

Exercise regularly: As for exercise, if your health allows, you should exercise daily in some form, even if it is only sit-ups or a fun activity like dancing. Exercise is generally best done as a steady enjoyable lifestyle rather than done excessively. This is because if over time you over do it and have to stop suddenly such as due to injury, the muscle you build up may turn into fat. We exercise about 4-6 days a week doing exercises such as yoga, lifting weights, and cardiovascular exercises including Argentine tango.

Exercise has many health and fitness benefits but losing weight is not always one of them. Exercise helps you lose weight mostly because it causes you to breathe more, and you lose most of your weight by breathing anyway with or without exercise. But here is the thing. Many people try to lose weight by mainly exercising but cannot make much progress because they eat too much. We hear that all the time: "I exercise a lot but can't lose any weight". They may lose 500 Calories with an hour or two of spin biking, and then afterwards in a few minutes gain it all back by drinking one smoothie with equal or greater Calories. Perhaps it is not an accident that many gyms have smoothie bars.

Exercise can help to burn Calories, but to lose weight you must also control how much you eat. So, if you are not losing the weight you want, whether you are exercising or not, guess what? You must be eating more Calories than you need to maintain your ideal weight, and you may not even know it.

Make the magic: You are now ready to try to make the magic. With our *Lowellie*™ Way, you could see the fruits of your labor: a leaner, stronger, and more energetic you. No need for short-term weight loss programs and useless dietary supplements. After about three months you should naturally crave correct food thereafter and not want the bad food that got you weight related issues in the first place. If you keep up with a healthy diet, you may not even crave bread nor do you need to have a "diet" anymore which makes it easier to continue your journey to the magic of losing weight. A possible reason for these three months may come as a surprise to you. Thanks to your hard-working metabolism, your body almost completely rebuilds/remodels itself every two to three months. Try the Lowellie™ Way for at least three months and see for yourself. What have you got to lose—the weight?

Keep the magic alive: With *Lowellie*™ Way your success often comes down to whether your body saves fat or burns fat, or whether it can make the burnable energy you need to perform your daily activities. Think of yourself as a magician that performs a hit magic show on the stage: eating the correct food in the correct amount. But, behind the scenes, you owe your success to your hard-working metabolism assistant that keeps the show prep down to, literally, the science. Your hard-working metabolism keeps the magic alive by making your body a fat burning machine. That fat burning machine can be capable of producing optimum energy for a healthier and more energetic you. With the magic alive, an occasional deviation does not kick you off the bandwagon. So, on occasion, you can have your bread and wine and eat it too!

Through experience and knowledge of fundamental mechanisms of how your body works and why what you eat matters, we explain what food you should eat or better yet what food you should not eat based on how you feel. For example, we do not eat bread or drink alcohol very much because intake of alcohol and/or bread causes an initial surge in blood sugar raising our insulin level, which saves fat and reduces energy level. There is a saying: "It is better to learn how to fish rather than be given a fish". So, let us go fishing.

Chapter 5: How Metabolism Creates Your Energy

You may have seen headlines like "Boost your metabolism" or "Try this high-metabolism diet to lose weight". Metabolism is more than how fast your body burns digested food as touted in articles with such headlines. Metabolism is the sum of all types of metabolic biochemistry reactions in your cells that maintain your life. To know what food you should eat, you should know how your metabolism works. We will examine what makes up your metabolism and how your metabolism works in terms of digesting the foods you eat to obtain food fuel for your cells to create the burnable energy you need.

5.1 Metabolism: A Sisyphean task

The "sciencey" word, metabolism, has acquired a meaning in popular speech, but metabolism is not just one thing. People talk about metabolism as meaning how fast your body burns the Calories in your food fuel, or how high your personal energy level is. That may be okay for health and fitness magazines and commercials with slogans such as "Boost your metabolism", or "Try this high-metabolism diet to lose weight". But physiologically metabolism really describes a sum of all types of metabolic biochemical reaction that goes on in your body. Maybe more importantly, it reconciles two conflicting chemical processes that are always simultaneously underway inside of you. These two conflicting chemical processes are the breakdown and removal of dead cells, and the production of new cells to replace the dead cells. Both processes require fuel from food—food fuel.

Energy measured in Calories in these food fuels is turned into a burnable energy in the form of adenosine triphosphate (ATP), a ubiquitous chemical in the body that can be burned in your cells to provide the primary fuel for your daily metabolic functions. ATP contains high-energy electrochemical bonds which, when split with the help of enzymes, release energy for use by all the body's metabolic systems that need burnable energy. For example, the muscles for movement, the liver for protein synthesis, and the brain for neural transmission, just to name a few.

Your body converts what you eat into ATP energy and raw materials through a never-ending series of reactions that are dedicated to doing two vital and contradictory things. One set of chemical reactions, catabolic reactions, destroys the reactants that you give them, reducing the big complex substances into molecular rubble. Another set of chemical reactions, anabolic reactions, reassembles that rubble and new material into new and bigger products that are put together again to make you. So, your body is constantly reinventing itself with never-ending loss and rebuilding.

Catabolic reactions break down bigger molecules, and in breaking their bonds, release the burnable energy you need to stay warm and move around and provide yourself with food fuel to build those polymers back up again. For example, digestion is also a form of catabolism that results in the breakdown of macronutrients into food fuels. Carbohydrates break down into monosaccharides also called simple sugars such as glucose (mainly), fructose, and galactose. Proteins in food are broken down to amino acids, and dietary fats are broken down to fatty acids and glycerol. Furthermore, fatty acids are broken down and converted to an alternate energy source called ketones or ketone bodies which we will explain in later chapters. Also, when cells in your body die, white blood cells digest the dead cells into food fuel that is reused and waste that is eliminated.

Anabolic reactions construct things and consume energy. These are the processes that take the small building blocks in your food and build them into bigger, more complex polymers that are used in your cells. For example, monosaccharide sugars, fatty acids, and amino acids are built back into carbohydrates, fats, and proteins respectively. Then, when you need new building blocks, or you need to release some burnable energy, those polymers in your body, or new ones in your food, get broken up by catabolic reactions.

Your metabolism is like trying to organize all your computer files, schedules, memos, photos, etc., only for the computer bits to degrade and corrupt them, then you need to start all over again. If you had backed up all your files before they were corrupted, you could at least access your raw data. In terms of your body, you have backed up energy stores/food fuel in the form of glycogen, a type of sugar molecule chain, in your liver and muscles, and triglycerides, a bound group of three fatty acids, in your fat cells. That is why you can build new cells after catabolism.

Like the Greek myth of Sisyphus, your metabolism is like pushing a large round heavy rock up the hill only to watching it fall back down. Your metabolism is a

Sisyphean task that works hard, but it is never finished. And the heavy rock that your metabolism is pushing uphill and falling back compares to nutrient molecules that your body is always breaking up and then rebuilding only to have them break apart again. And these nutrients, the materials that your body needs to build, maintain, and repair itself come in six major groups: water, vitamins, minerals, protein, carbohydrate, and fat. To put this in perspective, you break down and rebuild 1 to 2 percent of your muscle each day, almost completely rebuilding yourself every two to three months. Rebuilding a healthy-you has a lot do to with the correct food. Choosing a healthy diet from the correct food is like storing a correct backup of your computer files in a well-maintained computer. With a healthy diet from the correct food, your body can also be well-maintained, and access correctly backed up energy stores to reboot you!

And even though all of this is happening at the cellular level, the consequences could hardly be larger. Catabolic and anabolic reactions are where everything about digestive, endocrine, circulatory, and respiratory systems really starts to coalesce. Together all these types of metabolic biochemistry processes make up your metabolism.

5.2 What you are made of

If you weigh about 175 pounds (79 kilograms), most of that is water, but you cannot tell by looking since as organisms go, and unlike a jellyfish, you look solid. After water, the next largest fraction of you is protein, about sixteen percent. Protein is not just in your muscles, but also in things like the tiny sodium-potassium pumps in your nerve cells that control your nerve impulses. Protein also maintains your kidney's sodium-potassium balance, acid balance, blood pressure, steady cardiac contraction, and the hemoglobin which is a protein in your red blood cells. Protein in the form of enzymes drives the chemical reactions in all your 30 trillion cells. Some chemical reactions in the body take 78 million years to break down without an enzyme, and 18 milliseconds with the enzyme! So, without protein, life as we know it would not be possible. That is how important protein is for your body.

Another sixteen percent of you is fat, which you may be totally okay with, or want to get rid of some. Four percent of you is minerals, like the calcium and phosphorus in your bones and the iron in your blood. And, one percent is carbohydrates, most of which is either being consumed if you are going about your daily life, talking, and thinking, or is sitting around as glycogen waiting to be used. Although this one tiniest fraction of you that is carbohydrates ends up creating a large percentage of all the burnable energy you need, it is also *most responsible for your weight gain*, the blood sugar level, and blood sugar concentration.

But here is the thing: It is not like 175 pounds (79 kilograms) of food spontaneously formed your body. Instead, your body is constantly consuming food, extracting some of it to keep, burning some of it for energy, and getting rid of the rest. But even the stuff your body does hold on to does not last forever. Some of the chemicals that you absorb in your food eventually become a part of you, but enzymes wear out and membranes break down and DNA gets oxidized. So, they get discarded and then you need more of those chemicals to reconstruct the material that you have lost. As a result, over the course of your lifetime, your cells will synthesize somewhere between about 490-990 pounds (222-449 kilograms) of protein. That is like a small helicopter, a large bull, or a grand piano made of protein. And all the materials for the protein, fat, carbohydrates, and nucleic acids that make-up you come from food. Every organism must keep taking in and breaking down food to keep resupplying itself with the raw materials it needs to survive. In this manner, you almost completely rebuild yourself every two to three months. So, what you eat has a major impact on how successfully your body is regenerated.

5.3 All metabolism activities require ATP

All that activity requires burnable energy in the form of ATP, which you also gain from food. This burnable ATP is mainly from the one percent of you that is carbohydrates, although fat and protein can also contribute to making ATP based on availability of energy resources in the form of food fuels.

A main purpose of food is to get digested to provide food fuel for your cells. Mitochondria are special powerhouses of your cells which generate most of your ATP. Your body takes the Calories from these food fuels to your mitochondria, and the mitochondria catabolize these food fuels to generate burnable ATP. Think of mitochondria as the engine of your body. A car engine turns gas into mechanical energy. Similarly, mitochondria turn the Calories in food fuel into ATP.

The underlying process is remarkable. Your body uses ATP like a battery that can power your body's chemical reactions alternating between ATP and Adenosine Diphosphate (ADP) by losing or gaining one phosphorous group. Your body uses Calories from food fuel to convert the ADP to ATP so that the burnable energy is available to do needed work, and ATP is consumed to do the work becoming ADP again. That is how your body converts Calories from food fuel into burnable energy. Since you have about 30 trillion cells in your body that makes about 68 million ATPs per cell per second, roughly 2 million glucose molecules are needed per second for this. If not recycled, the human body would turn over the equivalent of its own weight in ATP daily, with ATP recycling to ADP and back again. Quite amazing!

Chapter 6: Why do you Gain Weight in the First Place?

There are several reasons why you gain weight instead of maintaining or losing weight. Normally, fat is burned by the brain signaling fat cells to release energy packages of fatty acid molecules to the bloodstream when needed. Your body cells, in the skeletal muscles, lungs, kidneys, liver, heart, and others, pick up these fatty acids from the fat cells. Your body cells then break them apart and use the energy stored in the bonds between the atoms to create ATP to execute their activities. This leaves many fat cells shrunken or empty. The body cells have a short lifespan so when they die, the body absorbs most of the empty cast and generally does not replace them. Over time, the body directly extracts the Calories from digested food into the body cells that need them instead of first storing the Calories in fat cells. As a result, the body readjusts by decreasing the number and size of fat cells, which subsequently improves baseline metabolism, decreases inflammation, treats disease, and prolongs lives.

If you maintain this situation over time, the body reabsorbs the extra empty fat cells and discards them as waste, leaving you leaner and healthier on multiple levels. Well, this is what is supposed to happen, if you have a healthy body operating in a fat burning state. But nowadays most people do not fall in the healthy category, and they may not even know why they get excess fat in the first place. Some primary reasons for gaining weight are as follows:

Reason 1: Because you eat more Calories than your body needs

"I eat healthy, but why do I gain weight," you might ask. As a basic principle, we describe losing weight as simply less Calories coming in than going out. Exercise helps to burn Calories, but not enough. To lose weight, you must watch how much you eat. If you eat more Calories than your body needs, the excess is converted to fat. Dietary fat, carbohydrates, and protein all convert to cellular fat if you eat more Calories than your body needs, albeit in a roundabout way. Within the intestinal cells the triglycerides (fat) are reassembled and then released into your blood stream along with ingested cholesterol in healthy "packages" of healthy proteins called chylomicrons. The body's tissues then remove the triglycerides from the circulating chylomicrons, either burning it for ATP energy or storing it as fat if you do not use them. The reassembled triglycerides are for most part stored in the muscle or fat cell tissue for later use. It is also possible for fat cells to take up glucose and amino acids, which have been absorbed into the bloodstream after a meal and convert those into fat molecules. Furthermore, when you eat both fat and carbohydrates, the carbohydrates, unlike fat, can only be stored in limited quantities, so the body is eager to use them for energy and stores the fat, so you get fat.

Reason 2: Because your body is designed to be energy efficient

To get better mileage in terms of your activities and more energy per unit of food fuel, your body chooses between Calories obtained from this food fuel. It is amazing, that your body has a winning strategy, it prefers the path of least resistance to produce energy, "When fighting on a hill, do not climb".

As such, to get better mileage from your activities, your body is designed to be energy efficient. Given a choice, a fat cell will grab the fat and store it rather than store the carbohydrates, because fat is so much easier to store, whereas you can only store a day or two of carbs. So, your body's first line of defense in maintaining energy is to break down carbohydrates, as well as glycogen, into simple glucose molecules and keep the fat. Your body uses the least number of Calories to store the most amount of energy, thus it can make you fat.

When it is turned into Calories, protein provides 4 Calories of energy for every gram of protein you consume. This is the same amount you will get from carbohydrates, but fat delivers 9 Calories per gram. Any extra Calories you consume above your ideal weight are stored as fat because fat is such a concentrated source of energy. The conversion of carbohydrates or protein into fat is 10 times less efficient than simply storing fat in a fat cell, but the body can do it. If you have 100 extra Calories in fat (about 11 grams) floating in your bloodstream, fat cells can store it using only 2.5 Calories of energy. On the other hand, if you have 100 extra Calories in glucose (about 25 grams) floating in your bloodstream, it takes 23 Calories of energy to convert the glucose into fat and then store it. So, your body chooses to spend less energy by storing the fat instead.

Storing fat in your fat cells is like pumping gas in your car. You fill up your gas tank with gas to run your car, similarly you fill up your cells with food fuel (fat / triglycerides) to run your body. The difference between your car and your body is that if you put too much fuel in your car tank it overflows, but if you put too much food fuel in your fat cell it overflows and multiplies, and you get more fat. Unless you burn it, the fat will most likely stay around your belly. However, you can outsmart your body by having a balanced diet of correct food and keeping your Calories within the Calories of your ideal weight. In this manner, you burn everything including the fat to get the ATP for all your cells that need them.

Reason 3: Because your microbiome is not balanced

There are myriad different types of cells contained in your body that are not human cells, but rather bacterial cells. Within your mouth, skin, and digestive tract live 10s (some say 100s) of trillions of different minute microbes. These are bacteria, viruses, molds, fungi, and protozoa. Your health may be as dependent on them as theirs is on you.

You host these microbes, and they provide many benefits to you the host in return. They rely on you to feed and house them, and you are also dependent on them. The largest quantity of these bacteria, called the gastrointestinal microbiome, reside in the normal human gastrointestinal tract. The major role your microbiome plays is to digest food and convert it into energy. They also contribute to gastrointestinal health and are defenders of your health. These good bacteria break down the food you cannot digest and pass the broken-down food into you. The good bacteria also battle with things you eat that could harm you, such as bad bacteria and plant proteins. While the good bacteria are in the majority you should be okay, but when the bad ones are controlling there is imbalance, "Houston we have a problem".

Depending on how your microbiome is balanced, you may crave good or bad food, with your appetite modified accordingly. One theory of why you desire certain foods is that your brain receives chemical signals from the bacteria in your gastrointestinal microbiome. The vagus nerve: the largest nerve coming from the brain to the gastrointestinal track, sends the chemical signals between the brain and the gastrointestinal track. Some of these chemical signals may depend on the needs of your microbiome. Healthy food develops more good bacteria (e.g., probiotics) which love to eat good food, while discouraging bad bacteria (e.g., pathogens) which love to eat bad food. Thus, you may crave good or bad food accordingly.

If you drive off the good bacteria, by taking antibiotics, etc., or letting the bad ones in, the bad bacteria may take over the vagus nerve communication path. The bad bacteria may then send chemical signals to your brain for bad food, making you crave the bad foods that they need. So, when you feel tired, sick, or overweight you know who to blame.

In contrast, if you keep your good bacteria, you may crave quality food instead. Quality food prevents the bad bacteria from promoting their food as your preferred food by preventing them from taking over the vagus nerve communication path. In this manner, good bacteria send their own chemical signal to your brain for good food. Accordingly, you crave the correct foods that you need, not what bad bacteria need. So, when you feel energetic, healthy or at your ideal weight you know who to thank.

To maintain a balanced population of gastrointestinal microbiome, in which the good bacteria outnumber the bad bacteria, you can eat the correct food such as fiber, and probiotic foods (e.g., yogurt, kefir, kimchi, and sauerkraut), and reduce the bad food. Examples of bad food include harmful plant proteins, and highly processed foods such as refined sugary foods, junk foods, and fast foods. Thus, you eliminate extra bad bacteria, and return the balance to your microbiome.

Remember we mentioned, if you keep up with a healthy diet, you may not even crave bread anymore? Miraculously, your body is, in effect, almost completely rebuilt every two to three months by replacement of dying cells throughout your body. If you eat the correct food, you most likely rebuild a healthier you, and consequently develop a healthy appetite—no more craving bad food.

Reason 4: Because your body is in a fat saving state

If, for any or all of the above reasons, your body ends up in a fat saving state, you can remedy the fat saving state by increasing fat burners, and reducing fat savers, as we explain in the next chapter. To get a feel for why fat savers and fat burners can play a major role in saving or losing fat, think of your body as an extraordinarily complex bio-logical machine comprising a bio-logical architecture. The bio-logical architecture may comprise: a network of bio-logical parts we call "organs", a central computer that we call the brain, and a metabolism as its overall operating system that generates ATP to operate your body. Your body, the bio-logical machine, produces at least one output for every input based on its present state. You intake oxygen and out comes CO_2. You eat sugar and insulin shows up. You eat protein and amino acids are formed. You eat fat, and your liver makes glucose. And, lo and behold, you eat more Calories than you need, and fat shows up, etc. Similarly, simply put, if you input fat savers, you save fat, and if you input fat burners you lose fat.

You can either operate your body with a fat saving metabolism using "cheap gas" containing fat savers, or with a fat burning metabolism using a "premium fuel" containing fat burners. The fat savers interrupt, or may even halt, ATP production, making you fat and tired. With fat burners, on the other hand, you not only lose fat, but also get more energetic. The good news is that the choice is yours. We choose the latter.

Chapter 7: Fat Savers and Fat Burners

To avoid repetition, we coin two terms: fat savers and fat burners. Fat savers decrease your energy and put your body in a fat saving state, so you get fat and tired. In contrast, fat burners increase your energy and put your body in a fat burning state, so you lose fat and gain more energy.

7.1 Fat savers

Fat savers comprise three major categories: anti-nutrients such as bad lectins, excess insulin, and stress.

Lectins: Swamp thing from the little shop of triffids

Most plants do not want to be eaten. Unlike in the movies though, they cannot chase you (Swamp Thing, Thing from another World, Day of the Triffids), or eat you (Little Shop of Horrors). They protect themselves by encasing and/or poisoning their edible parts. As such, most plants are your enemies, and they try to fill their tissue with toxic chemicals that can harm, sicken, and kill you if you eat them. You must cook many plants to destroy the toxins to make them edible. Alternatively, growers harvest immature plants before they develop their defenses such as asparagus which they harvest before it develops cellulose. The most abundant food from a plant is in the form of cellulose (e.g., wood), which despite being a polysaccharide comprising glucose sugar, is virtually indigestible even after cooking.

Fortunately, not all plants are always our enemies, and some plants do want to be eaten sometimes such as fruits that are ripened and want to be eaten so their seeds are spread around. The most effective way for plants to survive is to multiply quickly and in large numbers, so they generally waste little energy on defenses and focus more on growth. Toxins are usually a secondary defense but can still be a problem.

Lectins are a type of plant toxin. Most edible plants and animals comprise toxic substances such as lectins, but some of us have a tolerance for some of them such as gluten in bread. Furthermore, not all lectins are bad, and many are good for us, since like most animals we contain them ourselves. However, not everyone can digest every lectin containing food, for example, once again gluten.

Living things seek self-preservation, and lectins are a plant's defenses against insects and other herbivores. Lectins can paralyze insects that bite the plant. You might think you should not be worried about lectins since you are much larger than insects; however, you are still susceptible to the poisonous effect. Recall the infamous peanut allergies, a single peanut containing lectin has the potential to kill some people with such an allergy. Having said that, most people will not be paralyzed by most lectins immediately after consumption. Because of our comparatively large size and larger number of cells, any damaging effect may only be slow and long-term.

Lectins are a type of protein present in most plant and animal tissues that can bind to sugars and cell membranes, and make molecules stick together, which can affect cell-to-cell interaction. Lectins target and attach themselves to sugar molecules, primarily on the surface of the cells of organisms such as fungi, insects, and animals. Lectins also bind themselves to sialic acid, an acidic sugar molecule found in the intestines, in the brain, between nerve endings, in joints, and most bodily fluid, including the blood vessel lining of most creatures.

Because of these binding processes, lectins are sometime referred to as "sticky proteins". By sticking to these body parts, lectins may interrupt messaging between cells or otherwise cause toxic inflammatory reactions. For example, when lectin binds to sialic acid, one nerve may be unable to communicate its information to another nerve. Lectins also facilitate the attachment and binding of viruses and bacteria to their intended targets.

One reason some people get sick more often than others may be because they are more sensitive to lectins. These "sticky proteins" coat your intestinal tract, making it difficult to properly absorb micronutrients. While micronutrient loss due to lectins is an important concern, it is also important to understand other ways that lectins can negatively affect your health. To begin with, lectins make you fat in three unique ways: they effectively cause insulin resistance, can stimulate hunger, and may make the wall of your intestines leaky. Let us investigate how these three unique ways can cause weight gain:

First: They effectively cause insulin resistance. They impersonate insulin and sneak in and attach to receiving ports such as insulin receptors of fat cells, muscle cells and nerve cells. Once attached, these look-alike insulin impersonators may never detach and leave no room for real insulin to dock on the ports to guide delivery of sugar to the cells via glucose channels. In the case of fat cells insulin normally can bind to the insulin receptors and instruct the fat cells to make fat from glucose and detach itself when it is done. But lectins may permanently bind to the insulin receptors and instruct fat cells to make fat from glucose continuously.

As such, these insulin look-alikes not only cause fat cells to make more fat, but they also strain your ATP energy production. When these insulin look-alikes attach to the insulin receptors of muscle cells and nerve cells, they block delivery of sugar into these cells as well. So, these cells will not be able to generate the ATP you need. To add insult to the injury, in the case of muscle cells, the sugar is shunted instead to fat cells to make more fat, while the muscle starves and loses mass. The overall result is you get less muscle mass, more fat, and less energy.

One of these insulin look-alikes in bread is wheat germ agglutinin. Remember when we discussed the Lowellie™ Way, we said eliminate bread. Guess we could say we rest our case:)

Second: Lectins can also stimulate hunger and thus weight gain. Lectins can attach themselves to receptor sites for leptin, the hormone that tells your brain when you are full and block its effect. As a result, you become prone to overeating because you may never get the message that you are full and more of what you eat gets stored as body fat. If this is not enough, more fat is coming. Overeating exhausts your mitochondria, causing your muscle cells and nerve cells to reject sugar that they need to make ATP. Instead, your fat cells grab the extra sugar and double down on making more fat. We already told you about insulin look-alikes causing insulin resistance, here we are again, exhausted, overloaded, and unhappy mitochondria stop accepting sugar thus causing insulin resistance as well. So, whether you become resistant to insulin via insulin look-alikes, or by overeating, or both, the overall result is the same. You get less muscle mass, more fat, and less energy. But the good news is that you can fix that, as we will explain in the following chapters.

Third: When you eat food, it goes to your intestines, which convert the food into various forms of chemical compounds through the digestion process. Food containing bad lectins (e.g., wheat) may inflate the wall of your intestines and make the wall leaky and permeable. Intestinal permeability allows all sorts of bad things into your blood stream and the immune system goes wild as a result. For example, food is digested into small pieces of glucose, fatty acids, and amino acids that can be absorbed through the small intestine's walls. If they are released into your blood stream prematurely due to intestinal permeability, they may get attacked by your immune system as if they are foreign objects, thus causing inflammation. Plus, the belly starts collecting and storing food for the white blood cells that rush in to help destroy harmful substances to prevent illness. So, you get belly fat.

In food scarce ancient times, unbeknownst to them, people had a "lectin diet" to gain weight. Wheat became the preferred grain of the people in northern climates in part due to its uniquely small lectin known as wheat germ agglutinin, which is responsible for weight-gaining propensity. A "big belly" was a sign of affluence, and northerners gained and maintained weight by eating wheat.

Insulin: The fat saver—when your insulin goes high your waistline goes wide

In terms of metabolic biochemistry, insulin maintains life by keeping your blood sugar level regulated. Although the importance of insulin cannot be emphasized enough, insulin is also the main fat storage hormone in your body. The first key player to know when it comes to fat saving is enzyme lipoprotein lipase (LPL). LPL is a fat storer that can be activated by insulin. It makes triglycerides (a form of fat) and puts them in a fat cell for storage. Another important player is an enzyme hormone sensitive lipase (HSL) which lets that fat out if insulin allows it. When the insulin level is high, insulin does not allow fat out of fat cells, instead insulin interacts with LPL and HSL to make and store fat, as we will further explain below.

Glucose is a precious food fuel for all the cells in your body when it is present at normal levels as regulated by insulin. When you eat a candy bar your pancreas creates insulin to regulate it. A normal level of insulin causes the liver to convert more glucose into glycogen for short-term storage in a process called glycogenesis. Insulin also forces muscle and fat cells to take up glucose from the blood, thus decreasing blood sugar while producing ATP for your body to function. Once the cells have had their fill of glucose, the liver stores some of the excess for distribution between meals should blood glucose levels fall below a certain threshold—so far so good.

However, if you eat a lot of sugary candy bars your insulin level may increase considerably, and excess insulin commands fat saving. Excess insulin may play a key role in the development of high triglyceride levels because excess insulin may cause the liver to get saturated with glycogen and resist further conversion of glucose to glycogen. Instead, insulin activates enzyme LPL to use any leftover glucose, beyond what the liver can hold, to create fatty acids (e.g., triglycerides) that are converted into lipoproteins and exported from the liver into the bloodstream, so none is wasted. Insulin also orders all nearby fat cells to lock all their exits and not release any new energy into cells by blocking HSL. So, fat has a harder time getting out of the fat stores and the body starts storing fat in the fat cells and burning glucose instead. But when insulin goes too high and blocks cells from using glucose, good luck burning glucose too. Then what happens? Your waistline gets wider.

The title match between you and your waistline

In the ring are two fighters. One is you a former lightweight champion and the other is your waistline a current heavyweight champion. This is a match of you against your waistline who is fighting to keep its heavyweight title. You fight to change the waistline title to skinny one. Without any further delay, "Let's get ready to rumble!":

Round One: Waistline's strategy to win the fight is to convert all sugars to fat for itself and leave your cells powerless. To start the fight against you, your waistline counts on your cells to form an army of hormones to resist insulin and close their fuel receiving ports controlled by insulin receptors. Consequently, although there is enough insulin to unlock the cells, the receiving ports are under siege and heavily guarded. And thus, the insulin and the sugar cargo are turned away at the receiving ports and their controlling insulin receptors. As good defensive skills are just as important as good attacking skills, insulin decides to suffer a loss to the waistline, but lives to fight on your side for another round. Giving in to the waistline's demands, insulin instructs the enzyme LPL to make fat cells turn all the sugar into more fat and store them in the waistline instead of giving them to your cells to produce ATP. Despite enough food in the sugar cargo, cells remain hungry. The waistline is smiling and toying with you, trying to give the fans (fat cells) their money's worth and make a show of it while making you look badly outmatched. At the same time, to add insult to injury, the waistline sends a false hunger signal ghrelin, a hunger hormone, to trick the brain to get more sugar. "Where is my sugar?", the waistline asks.

This is a double combination that snaps you back into a corner. The bell rings, and the waistline wins round one.

Round Two: The false hunger signal ghrelin, by which your waistline snaped you back into a corner in round one, keeps fooling the brain that there is excess insulin and that your cells are starving for glucose. So, in response, your brain increases your appetite. Your brain creates cravings for carbohydrates and signals your body to store fat by ordering carbohydrates to be burned for energy rather than body fat. The false hunger signal from ghrelin continues to influence insulin secretion and vice versa, stimulates appetite, increases food intake, and promotes fat storage. This makes your body too readily store food in the form of fat as if you need to prepare for a storm. As such, once the food is consumed, insulin continually signals the body to store the energy from the food in the form of fat. So, your waistline wins again, but insulin lives to fight along your side another round.

Round Three: To win the fight, at some point your brain should wise up and figure out that it cannot trust the waistline, so it asks for a backup troop of leptins, a satiety hormone, to decrease your appetite. But here is the thing, your waistline outmatched you preemptively in this round too when it took advantage of your resistance to insulin in the first round. The waistline figured out that your communication line with leptin was terminated, when in round two, it blocked glucose from getting into the cell to produce the ATP power that your brain needs for communication with leptin. Instead, as sneakily planned, the waistline spoofs the communication line and sends its own signal ghrelin to deceive your brain again to get more sugar. So, while you eat more, your fat cells turn sugar into more fat and deposit them into the waistline account instead of generating the ATP you need. So, you get tired, and your waistline gets fat and happy. Your waistline wins again.

You win, the GRAND FINALE: Enough is enough. Fool me once, shame on you; fool me three-times, shame on me. The audience (your cells) cheers… "You can do it! You've got the power! The insulin, get the insulin in check!!!"

You take over to remove the fat title from your waistline. It is time to show the waistline who is outmatched—you or your waistline? You stop eating too much "candy" such as sugar, honey, fruits, fruit juice, alcohol, and other carbohydrate-rich foods. So, your pancreas stops producing too much insulin preventing the insulin from directing the enzyme LPL to make more fat. The waistline gets a first knock down—you get a first win. The waistline's playful attitude is gone… no more toying with you.

As the fight continues, cells' insulin receptors receive insulin, unlocking and drawing glucose into themselves to make ATP, thus enabling the brain's communication with leptins to reduce your appetite, instead of making fat cells turn sugar into more fat. The waistline gets a second knock down, and you get a win again. You outwit your waistline by eating more protein during the fight. With an adequate amount of protein, your waistline can no longer sabotage your brain's communication link to trick you to eat more. Your brain wises up, not afraid of getting right in the middle of the action, it does not accept any more false-hunger signals, so you eat less and lose weight automatically and without hunger. You win again.

Who is outmatched now? Tired of winning yet? If not, here is another one: the waistline is taking a beating, so give it the knockout punch—increase your insulin receptors by exercising regularly. Eight -- Nine -- Ten -- the fight is over. At the fourth and final round, the waistline takes the defeat and gives up its heavyweight title for a skinny one. How is this for an overmatch?

And you go for better and skinnier things, yeah, you are on a role. Keep it coming. Here is one for the road: refer to your QCC to maintain your Calories within the Calories of your ideal weight for about 3-4 months. After that, your body is most likely rebuilt with correct food, and you are familiar with nutrition and Calorie contents of the food you eat. So, you may not need to precisely count every Calorie anymore, nor should you be worried about a high insulin level, or leptin supplements. Your waistline gets a long-term skinny title, and you keep winning!

Stress

Stress releases the main stress hormone cortisol. Cortisol is a double-edged sword. Secreted by the adrenal glands, cortisol has several jobs essential to life including raising blood sugar, contributing to fat burning, and is even an anti-inflammatory in small doses. Yet, like insulin, when your body has cortisol in too-high doses, the cortisol can cause an increase in body fat, induce food cravings, contribute to inflammation, slow the metabolism by affecting thyroid hormone levels, and make you more insulin resistant.

So, it is not fair to only blame insulin for making your waistline bigger. Insulin and stress are the absolute worst combination, and a combination of insulin and cortisol from stress can operate in many ways. For example, the storage and release of fat can both be affected by insulin and cortisol. When the two are elevated together, it makes storing fat easier and burning fat harder. Furthermore, the insulin issue does not begin and end at storing fat, and the cortisol issue does not begin and end at stress. How these hormones uniquely interact in your body really tell a bigger story.

It's not that these hormones have different effects or varying intense effects, it also depends on which other hormones are also present. Some of these hormones, in combination, make managing your body composition much harder. When it comes to fat saving or losing, a whole host of hormones and enzymes play in a symphony orchestra of your metabolism conducted mostly but not only by the hormones insulin and cortisol. For example, whether you lose or gain fat depends on how the insulin and cortisol interact with each other and the rest of the orchestra which is mainly LPL and HSL enzymes. When cortisol and insulin are around together, the combination causes an exaggerated effect on LPL (fat storing) where insulin hinders HSL overriding cortisol trying to release fat for burning. Normally, during short periods of not eating such as during night, between meals, and short duration high-intensity exercise, cortisol will turn on the HSL enzyme triggering fat release. Cortisol does this with help from growth hormones and adrenaline, but chronically elevated cortisol can also make you more insulin resistant, blocking fat release.

But the good news is that cortisol and/or insulin are only the conductors in the orchestra and can only conduct the music you, the composer, write for them. So, it is up to you to write relaxing music for the orchestra by reducing your stress level through working less, dancing more, exercising regularly, and eating correct food-for-thoughts as we explain in Chapter 12.

7.2 Fat burners

Fat burners comprise protein to control your appetite, happy thoughts to reduce your stress, and oxygen to burn the fat.

Eating more protein to lose weight!

Protein makes you lose weight, even without conscious Calorie restriction because protein works on both sides of the "Calories in vs. Calories out" equation, it reduces Calories in and boosts Calories out. However, losing weight is not the most important factor. Keeping it off in the long-term is what really counts. Protein does not just help you lose weight; it can also help prevent you from gaining weight in the first place. Many people can go on "a diet" and lose weight, but most end up gaining the weight back.

Protein is the easiest, simplest, and most delicious way to lose weight. Your weight is actively regulated by your brain particularly in an area called the hypothalamus. For your brain to determine when and how much to eat, it processes multiple different types of information. Some of the most important signals to the brain are hormones that change in response to feeding. Protein changes the levels of these weight regulating hormones, and protein can help you lose weight and prevent you from gaining weight in the first place because protein can reduce hunger and appetite via several different mechanisms.

Appetite regulator

A higher protein intake increases levels of a suite of appetite-reducing hormones, while reducing levels of the only known hunger-stimulant hormone ghrelin. A higher protein intake that is generally above 16% of your daily Caloric intake also boosts several satiety hormones such as leptin which inhibit appetite stimulation.   These appetite-reducing, hunger-stimulant and satiety hormones are collectively referred to as appetite modulators. Higher protein intake increasing the appetite-reducing hormones leads to a major reduction in hunger and is one of the main reasons that protein helps you lose weight. Thus, protein can make you eat fewer Calories automatically without the need to take any appetite control supplements.

In Chapter 6, we mentioned one of the reasons that you gain weight is because your body is designed to be energy efficient. Given a choice, your body prefers to burn the Calories from carbs because they are the most efficient to burn, and stores fat because fat is the more concentrated and more taxing to burn. Beware that your waistline is always on watch to regain its heavyweight title: the one that you changed to a skinny title in the title match between you and your waistline. So, when you store the fat at the expense of burning excess carbs instead, your waistline is happy to keep the fat for you. Your waistline never quits trying to defeat you, if push comes to shove, it does not even hesitate to go to the lengths of resistance to insulin to make you powerless. However, as you did in the title match between you and your waistline, you can outwit your waistline by eating more protein. With an adequate amount of protein, your waistline cannot sabotage your brain's communication link to trick you to eat more. Instead, your brain can communicate via the appetite modulators to signal whether you had enough food or not, and thus regulate your food intake accordingly. So, you can avoid the excess carbs, and burn the fat instead, disappointing the waistline!

Facilitating communication with appetite modulators such as leptins is not the only way that protein reduces your appetite. Protein also reduces your appetite because it keeps you fuller for longer. Amino acids are chemically like glucose except that they contain nitrogen. This means that even after protein is digested into amino acids, they must go through more steps to have the nitrogen removed. Once the nitrogen is gone, the amino acids are converted into glucose or fatty acids. Due to the extra steps, protein provides a slower but longer-lasting source of energy (Calories) than carbohydrates, so it keeps you fuller for longer. That is why you get less hungry with more protein consumption.

As a bonus, this extra step also costs you Calories. About 30 percent of protein Calories provided by protein is needed to digest protein itself to get rid of the excess nitrogen. This means that 30 percent of protein Calories are not available to be converted to fat or carbs for storage. So, 100 Calories of protein would end up as about 70 Calories when all digestion is done. In comparison, fat loses only 2 percent from this effect, so 100 Calories of fat would end up as fully 98 Calories. Put simply, high-protein diets have a metabolic advantage. Protein Calories are less fattening than Calories from carbs and fat because protein takes more energy to metabolize. Food labels generally show you the Calories in protein without considering this, so unbeknownst to you, you end up eating 30 percent less protein Calories than you may have accounted for!

Keep the muscles, lose the fat

Weight loss does not always equal fat loss. When you lose weight, muscle mass tends to be reduced as well. However, what you really want to lose is body fat, both subcutaneous fat (under the skin), and visceral fat (around organs). Losing muscle is a side effect of weight loss that most people do not want. A high protein intake also helps to build and preserve muscle mass, the muscle mass also burning a small number of Calories around the clock. So, people who want to hold on to muscle that they have already built may need to increase their protein intake when losing body fat, because a high protein intake can help prevent the muscle loss that usually occurs when dieting.

Protein can also increase your metabolic rate. Metabolic rate is the rate at which your metabolism does every metabolic biochemical reaction in your body. Another side effect of losing weight is that the metabolic rate tends to decrease partly because concentration of appetite control hormones such as leptin is reduced in the blood. So, you end up burning fewer Calories than you did before you lost the weight. This is often referred to as "starvation mode" and can amount to several hundred fewer Calories burned each day. Eating plenty of protein (about 25%-30% Calorie intake) can reduce muscle loss, which should help keep your metabolic rate higher as you lose body fat. More protein can help you gain muscle and strength because muscles are made largely of protein.

How to get more protein in your diet?

Increasing your protein intake is simple. Just eat more protein-rich foods. Animal foods are generally high in protein, with all the essential amino acids that you need. The best sources of protein are meat, fish, eggs and dairy products. Some plants are high in protein such as legumes, tree nuts, and nut butters, but you may need to consume more Calories to get the same amount of protein compared to animal products. Animal products generally have a higher protein concentration than plants.

If you are on a low-carb diet, you can choose fattier cuts of meat because normally carbs get burned first and fat gets stored around your belly. If you are not on a low-carb diet, then try to include lean meats as much as possible. This makes it easier to keep protein high without getting too many Calories. Although we prefer avoiding most diet products, we can make an exception of a protein supplement if you struggle to reach your protein goals. Protein supplements have been shown to have numerous benefits including increased weight loss; however, most people do not really need protein supplements though they can be useful for athletes and bodybuilders.

Even though eating more protein is simple when you think about it, integrating this into your life and nutrition plan can be difficult. We eat a variety of correct foods with high protein content such as meat, tree nuts, legumes, and dairy products; plus, a variety of correct fruits and vegetables with vitamin A and D. The presence of vitamin A and D is a requirement for the synthesis of keratin, the type of protein that makes up your hair, skin, and nails. For vitamin A, we generally have carrots, persimmons, celery, lettuce, and spinach. We can get vitamin D from tuna, salmon, milk, mushrooms, eggs, and sunlight. However, with these foods it is too easy to eat way more protein than you need. In the Lowellie™ Way, we choose the high side of protein intake spread between 3-5 meals per day based on our goals such as losing weight, gaining muscle, and just staying healthy. In Chapter 10 we will discuss how much protein may be too much and show you how you can calculate your protein intake based on your goals.

Generally, if you are just a healthy person trying to stay healthy, then simply eating quality protein with most of your meals (along with nutritious plant foods) should bring your intake into an optimal range. Although there may not be a need for most people to track their protein intake, it may be a good idea to know how much protein is in the food you eat anyway. You can do this by using a Calorie/nutrition tracker such as your QCC in the beginning of your diet. Weigh and measure everything you eat to make sure that you are hitting your protein targets. You need to do this for about two to three months only, but it is important in the beginning until you get a good idea of what a high-protein diet looks like for you.

No free lunch, Calories still count

When it comes to fat loss and a better-looking you, protein is the king of nutrients. You can generally benefit from a higher intake of protein in your diet without significantly affecting or limiting other aspects of your diet. This is particularly appealing because most high-protein foods also taste good. Eating more of them is easy and satisfying. A high-protein diet can also be an effective obesity prevention strategy, not something that you just use temporarily to lose fat. By increasing your relative protein intake, you may tip the "Calories in vs. Calories out" balance in your favor. Over months, years or decades, the difference in your waistline could be huge. Bear in mind that although protein can reduce hunger, boost metabolism, and keep you fuller for longer, you still may not lose weight if you do not eat fewer Calories than you burn. Calories still count, albeit protein Calories count 30 percent less than what may be on the food labels as we explained above.

Happy thoughts

Happiness is essential to good physical health as well as mental health. Your mind is at least the sum of your thoughts, and your physical body is a representation of your thoughts through the choices you make. After all, your body is not many years old! Your body is only months old, as some say about 98 percent of the cells in your body were probably replaced within the last few months! Happy thoughts block the negative thoughts that interfere with your body's natural healing mechanism, allowing your body to regenerate new cells for a healthier and happier you. You can change your body by changing your thoughts. You are what you think!

When speaking about willpower and happiness you may have heard people say: "It is all up here," pointing to their brain. It is literally true by virtue of happy neurotransmitters. Neurotransmitters are chemicals that help to carry signals between brain cells, aka neurons. Happiness comes from happy thoughts, happy thoughts come from happy neurotransmitters. Happy neurotransmitters can be activated by correct food-for-thoughts, which we define as a combination of correct food and exercise. Neurons release happy neurotransmitters into synapses to communicate with other neurons. While it is not known exactly how many neurotransmitters exist, scientists have identified more than 100 of these chemical messengers.

Endorphins, oxytocin, serotonin, and dopamine are just a few of the major neurotransmitters also known as happiness hormones that can supply happy thoughts. They act as neurotransmitters, but they are also considered hormones since they can carry messages throughout the nervous system, not just the brain. Increasing the level of these happy neurotransmitters in your nervous system transmits happy thoughts to your brain. Basically, you can be on brain drugs without the risk of drug addiction. Have you had a feeling of not wanting to do anything from time to time? If you wonder why, it is the work of your not so happy neurotransmitters. To activate happy neurotransmitters to transmit happy thoughts, you can eat the correct food-for-thoughts as we will discuss in Chapter 12.

With happy thoughts comes joy, and with joy comes an increase in available ATP energy. The increase in ATP increases desire to do more exercise, more exercise may reduce depression, and reduced depression reduces your desire to overeat to manage your emotions. Thus, you happily lose weight and that may be addictive.

Every breath you take will be shrinking you

When you lose weight, where does it go? Turns out, most of it is exhaled. This explains why exercise helps people lose weight, it speeds up breathing. Glucose plus oxygen produces carbon dioxide (CO_2), water, and energy. Lungs supply oxygen to the oxygen-depleted blood received from the heart and exhale CO_2 to remove waste, and thus we lose weight. By breathing more, you take more oxygen to the cells and burn more glucose and/or fat to create more immediate ATP energy. Since glucose plus oxygen produces CO_2 as an output, you lose most of your weight by breathing. This is a compelling reason for exercise.

For example, to burn 22 pounds (10 kilograms) of fat, a person needs to inhale 64 pounds (29 kilograms) of oxygen. Later we will tell you how many breaths and how many days it takes to lose 64 pounds (29 kilograms). The carbon you breathe out as CO_2 comes from the carbon in the food you eat. The food and drink you eat can be broken (metabolized) via enzymes into carbon compounds to produce energy. The carbohydrates, fat, and proteins you consume, are eventually converted by several different biochemical pathways in the body to glucose. Glucose plus oxygen produces CO_2, water and ATP energy. You use the energy of the ATP molecules, and the CO_2 molecules are dissolved in the blood, carried to the lungs by the circulation, and breathed out as gas. So, you lose weight.

Like other things in life, breathing is not that simple

What you breathe in is far from pure oxygen, it is roughly by volume 78 percent nitrogen, 21 percent oxygen, 1 percent argon and 0.04 percent CO_2, plus some water and other trace gases. The gases you exhale have roughly the same percent of nitrogen and argon, but you reduce the oxygen to 15 to 18 percent to produce and exhale 4 to 5 percent CO_2.

Some misconceptions about how humans lose weight may exist among some people. Some believe that fat is converted to energy or heat, which would violate the law of conservation of mass. Rather, fat does not simply "turn into" energy or heat, when consumed, it is broken down, oxidized, and excreted. In reality as we explained above, the body stores the excess protein or carbs in a person's diet in the form of fat in fat cells specifically as triglyceride molecules, which comprise three kinds of atoms: carbon, hydrogen and oxygen. The three elements make up the basic building blocks of living matter, including carbohydrates and fat. Breathing increases oxygen, oxygen combines with the carbon in the fat, and the carbon is exhaled out in the form of CO_2. You lose most of your weight by exhaling the CO_2 that used to be fat, that is by breathing.

The more breaths you take, the more carbon you lose. And you also lose a little weight just sitting on the couch watching TV, or even while you are asleep. Unfortunately, general living and eating easily compensates for this loss, and it does not alter the depressing fact that one pound of body weight equals 3,500 Calories. For people to lose weight, their triglycerides are broken up through oxidation in the body into the building blocks comprising carbon, hydrogen, and oxygen. When a triglyceride fat is oxidized (or "burned up"), the process consumes many molecules of oxygen while producing CO_2 and water as waste products. The good news is that you do not need to memorize complicated biochemistry to lose weight. Just breath more.

How many breaths does it take to lose a pound?!

As we mentioned above, to burn 22 pounds (10 kilograms) of fat, a person needs to inhale 64 pounds (29 kilograms) of oxygen. The chemical process of burning that fat will produce 62 pounds (28 kilograms) of CO_2 and 24 pounds (11 kilograms) of water. The average human exhales about 2.3 pounds (1 kilogram) of CO_2 on an average day in a sedentary breathing. The quantity of CO_2 depends on your activity level. A person engaged in vigorous exercise produces up to eight times as much CO_2 as his sedentary state. You might wonder about how many Calories per breath you may lose. That is an easy one, since the answers are readily available. It takes about 0.067 Calories per breath and 51,840 breaths to lose about one pound with 3500 Calories per pound.

You can only breathe so many times a day. At rest, you breathe around 12 times a minute or 17,280 times a day, and each one expels an average of 10 milligrams of carbon which is roughly 0.38 pounds (172.8 grams) per day. As such, you are going to lose roughly 0.38 pounds (172.8 grams) in a day with no exercise. In this manner, if you just breath for 3 days and do not eat anything you would lose about 0.5 kilogram or one pound (1.14 pounds=3.0x0.38 pounds/day)! That is, it takes about 51,840 (3x17,280) breaths to lose about one pound. So, as we promised to tell you, it would take 192 days and

3,317,760 breaths to lose 64 pounds (29 kilograms), assuming minimal food intake and you have enough weight to lose (Don't try this at home!).

7.3 The secret to weight loss remains the same

Don't underestimate the frightening power of, for example, a small muffin vs. an hour of exercise. At rest, you may exhale just 10 mg (0.067 Calories) of carbon with each breath. Even after an entire day, if you only sit, sleep, and do light activities, you may exhale about 173 grams (1158 Calories) of carbon. One 100 grams muffin (350 Calories) can restore 30 percent of what was lost.

On the other hand, replacing one hour of rest with exercise such as jogging, may remove only an additional 40 grams (1.4 oz) of carbon (i.e., about 360 Calories from fat carbon) from the body. So, the advice remains the same, losing weight requires unlocking the carbon stored in fat cells, thus reinforcing that often-heard refrain of "eat less, move more". Even if one traces the fate of all the atoms in the body, the secret to weight loss remains the same: either eat less carbon, or exercise more to remove extra carbon from your body, or both.

The good news is that over time by maximizing the fat burners and minimizing the fat savers you can build/rebuild a fat burning state for your body, where you may not even have to diet anymore! As in a vehicle that needs premium fuel to run optimally with minimum pollution, your body needs correct food to generate optimal burnable energy to run on. After all, creating burnable energy is what makes life possible, and creating an optimal burnable energy makes life not only possible but also more enjoyable! So, let us get to it.

Chapter 8: A More Energetic You

I t is not enough to keep an ideal weight if all you can do is sit on your couch and not move because you have no energy. If you use your food fuel more efficiently you should be more energetic than you were before. To use your food fuel more efficiently and do as much or more with less fuel, it is useful to know how your body uses your food fuel, and how optimizing your choice of food can give you more energy.

8.1 ATP energy in your body

ATP energy makes life possible and is your primary source of energy. Simply put, you eat to generate ATP through your metabolism. ATP can be generated either with the use of oxygen known as aerobic metabolism or without the use of oxygen by anaerobic metabolism. Anaerobic metabolism generally occurs during fast activities (e.g., during quick weightlifting, sprinting, or cycling) where there is no time to circulate significant oxygen to the muscles. Aerobic metabolism generally occurs during prolonged slow activities (e.g., sitting, walking, running, or cycling with sustained effort) where there is time to circulate oxygen to the muscles. Anaerobic metabolism occurs in the intra-cellular fluid inside muscle cells, and aerobic metabolism takes place in the mitochondrion of the cell.

Glucose (sugar) is the primary food fuel for both anaerobic and aerobic metabolism to produce ATP. The food fuel for anaerobic and aerobic metabolism will change depending on the amount of nutrients available and the type of metabolism. Glucose may come from blood glucose which is from dietary carbohydrates, protein, liver glycogen and glucose synthesis, or muscle glycogen.

Anaerobic metabolism uses glucose as its only food fuel and produces pyruvic acid and lactic acid which cause muscle fatigue. Muscles have a large glycogen storage (1200 kcal) which is about three-fourths of all the glycogen in the body. This glycogen is readily converted into glucose for use within muscle cells via anaerobic metabolism if not enough oxygen is available.

Aerobic metabolism generates ATP by burning glucose made from four basic food fuels: carbohydrates, protein, fatty acids, and ketones. Carbohydrates are the most important energy source, but in cases where carbohydrates have been depleted, the body can utilize protein, fats, and ketones in lieu of carbohydrates to generate ATP.

Although protein is not considered a major energy source, small amounts of amino acids from protein may be converted into ATP via aerobic metabolism. Or, if your diet does not meet nutrient needs or you are involved in long endurance exercises, amino acids from protein may be used to make glucose while you are resting or doing an activity.

Fatty acids are stored as triglycerides in muscles, but about 90 percent of stored triglycerides is found in fat cells. Many different cells such as cardiac muscle cells, kidney cells, liver cells and skeleton muscle cells use fatty acids for ATP production aerobically if enough oxygen is available. Indeed, fatty acids are the main source of ATP generated by mitochondria in skeletal muscle during rest and mild-intensity exercise. As exercise intensity increases oxygen becomes more available and aerobic oxidation of glucose takes place in mitochondria surpassing fatty acid oxidation. Yes, you could lose weight while sitting if you don't eat that cookie.

Ketones are a desirable method of generating ATP. In diet discussions, the term ketone is often used to refer to ketone bodies which are technically a subset of ketones. Ketones are made by your liver from fatty acids released from your fat cells when you are not getting enough energy from glucose. The most commonly known way to increase ketones in your body is by putting your body into a state of ketosis, which we will discuss in relation to low-carb diets and more specifically the Ketogenic diet in later chapters.

Most ATP production takes place in the mitochondria of your cells. Through breathing you give your cells the oxygen they need to burn ATP. ATP powers the muscles you need to move and breathe. Walking, thinking, working out, and moving your eyes to read these words all happens because your mitochondria are hidden away in your cells right now cranking out ATP. Producing and recycling the equivalent of your body weight over the course of the day. Think of ATP as your energy currency generated by the mitochondria treasury department of your body. Perhaps this is where the phrase "Your health is your wealth." came from.

8.2 How much energy do you need?

You need energy enough to maintain your ideal weight unless you are planning to lose or gain weight. The amount of daily energy your body requires depends on how much energy from food (Calories) you require per day to generate enough ATP to fuel your activities and to make all the supporting materials your body needs.

Your body is a bio-logical machine albeit an extraordinarily complex one and like any machine it requires energy to run. For example, if you require about 2,500 Calories per day to generate enough ATP to fuel your activities and to make all the supporting materials your body needs, eat about 2,500 Calories per day and your weight will remain unchanged. Chow down on 4,000 Calories per day, and 2,500 will be used to support all your biological needs, and much of the remaining excess 1,500 Calories will be converted to fat as storage for future use. Munch only enough to bring 1,000 Calories a day (only an example not a recommendation), and your body will convert the energy stored in your fat reserves to manufacture enough ATP to fill the 1,500 Calorie deficit. Bingo! You lose weight.

It all seems under control! In a healthy world your metabolism works hard to take the Calories you eat to your mitochondria to turn it into burnable ATP. But what if your mitochondria are not working properly? Are your cells receiving the food fuel you think you are providing, or do you just think they are? What if there is a mismatch between the food fuel and the ability of your mitochondria to handle it? What if you overwork your mitochondria? Can they still give you the ATP you need, or do they give up? If your mitochondria are overworked what happens to your body? How can you optimize your ATP production to get a more energetic you? We will give our answers to these questions in this chapter.

8.3 Better Mitochondria = More ATP

Your mitochondria not only provide ATP via cellular energy production they also play a central role in the aging process, brain function, heart function, immune system function, skeletal muscle strength, and more. Amazingly enough, a person will typically use the equivalent of his or her body weight in internally recycling ATP over the course of a day!

You want your mitochondria to be strong for general health reasons. Furthermore, mitochondrial dysfunction may be linked to cardiovascular diseases (CVDs), increased cell death, cellular aging, Alzheimer's disease, neurodegenerative diseases, shortened telomeres aging, DNA damage, etc. You lose mitochondrial function as you age, which may contribute to muscle loss, fat gain, decreased cognitive function, and fatigue. One theory of aging is that your mitochondria become less efficient over time and start producing increasing amounts of damaging free radicals, especially in mitochondria rich parts of your body such as your brain, muscles, and heart.

However, you do not have to resign yourself to declining mitochondria. The good news is that by making your mitochondria function in a fat burning state running on a premium food fuel, you can produce maximum burnable energy for your body. The result should be a more energetic and happier you. In the fat burning state: a state in which your body creates ample ATP, you can grow brand new happy mitochondria, and make the not-so-happy ones you already have more efficient. With the right habits, comprising a balanced diet of correct food and exercise, you can create and maintain a fat burning state to fix dysfunctional mitochondria and build strong shiny new ones.

As we mentioned in Chapter 5, choosing a healthy diet from correct food is like storing a correct backup of your computer files. Your body at least has access to backed up energy stores to remodel and reboot itself with correct information each time it loses some. Thus, your body can build brand new shiny mitochondria each time it loses some. So, why do mitochondria become unhappy? Let us explore the happy ones first before exploring the unhappy ones.

8.4 Happy Mitochondria = More energetic you

Mitochondria are happy when your body is in a fat burning state: a state in which they are not overloaded with a lot of incorrect food. Happy mitochondria function efficiently to convert food fuel to optimum ATP energy. Before we tell you how the same conversion can be obstructed with unhappy mitochondria overloaded with incorrect food, let us look at how mitochondria convert fat and sugar (glucose) to ATP when they are happy in the first place:

As for converting fat to ATP: Normally, in response to a need for ATP energy, a hormone signal (lipase) is sent to the fat cells to release stored fat. In response to fat cells receiving the hormone signal, your pancreas secretes the enzyme lipoprotein lipase (LPL), breaking up the reassembled triglycerides into their parts, glycerol and essential fatty acids, again. Fatty acids and glycerol are then released from triglycerides stored in fat cells into your blood, and travel towards the liver and other organs and tissues through the body and into mitochondria to generate ATP.

As for converting sugar to ATP: Normally, when you eat sugar, your pancreas secretes insulin to escort delivery of sugar into mitochondria throughout your body, where sugar is converted by the mitochondria into ATP.

So far so good. But not so fast.

8.5 Unhappy mitochondria **give up**

Mitochondria become unhappy when they are in a fat saving state. In a fat saving state, mitochondria become overburdened by work when you overload them with too much incorrect food. For example, too much sugar and/or fat may overburden the mitochondria. The mitochondria will process what it can, but like trying to put too much gas in your car, when the tank is full, the fuel spills out. Thus, cells block entry of excessive sugar, and fat into mitochondria. As we mentioned in Chapter 7, substances like lectins, may also block the intake of nutrients including sugar and fat into mitochondria. And both may occur, where sugar and/or fat overflows the cell because it is excessive, and because entry is blocked.

In cells with unhappy mitochondria, excess sugar and/or fat are not converted to ATP, and the excess overflows the cell and goes through the blood stream to fat cells for storage.

When you eat sugar or protein, your pancreas secretes insulin to facilitate sugar delivery into mitochondria. If, however, mitochondria are overworked and stressed trying to handle an excessive number of Calories that have been eaten, or cells have been blocked by lectins, cells refuse to accept the extra workload, and block insulin reception. The engine of your cell is broken. The ATP production is impaired, and your cells start a power outage.

In this situation, the insulin that controls delivery of sugar has nowhere to dock at cells' insulin receptors, so there is no "bell" to ring to alert the cells that sugar is coming. Thus, the cells' insulin-controlled channels are unaware of incoming sugar and do not open for receiving sugar. Instead, the sugar is dumped into fat cells, which gives an opportunity to your tenacious waistline to get ready for a re-match of the fight it lost to you in Chapter 7. Insulin instructs the enzyme LPL to make fat cells turn sugar into more fat and to store it instead of taking sugar into the mitochondria to make ATP. Remember once upon a time, when your mitochondria were happy, the very same enzyme LPL worked for you to release the fat into happy mitochondria to generate ATP. Now that your mitochondria are not-so-happy, the enzyme LPL works against you, and stores the fat instead of releasing it to your cells to burn. As a result, no matter how much sugar or fat you eat, your cells cannot generate enough ATP.

There are other problems caused by unhappy mitochondria. Your brain is the CEO of your body, sitting in the ivory tower of executive offices and has no idea what the workers' situation is "on the factory floor". The company is going broke "Somebody do something, produce or find some sugar, so I can generate some currency," the CEO keeps asking. But overloaded mitochondria have left the floor or cut back work. Same with your immune system, they cut back work too and stop guarding and watching the premises, leaving doors open for the bad guys (e.g., foreign viruses, bacteria, and cancer cells) to jump in and eat all that extra sugar that is lying around for taking. Your mitochondria give up under this kind of stress and tension, and your energy comes to a stop. While you have lots of fuel to burn, the engine of your cell is in power outage and cannot run to burn the fuel you provide, instead your fat cells store the fuel as fat. And you know the rest, you get fat and tired.

8.6 Sugar-sugar everywhere but you can't use it

A comprehensive explanation, without oversimplifying the science, of how unhappy mitochondria can affect your entire body would be outside the scope of this book. So as representative examples we explain what may happen to the high performer skeleton muscles and brain if mitochondria give up and do not accept sugar anymore.

Starving Skeleton muscles

The source of energy that is used to power contraction in working muscles is ATP. The major fuels for muscles to make ATP are glucose (sugar), fatty acids, and ketones. Indeed, fatty acids are the main source of food fuels for making ATP in skeletal muscle during rest and mild-intensity exercise. As exercise intensity increases, glucose oxidation surpasses fatty acid oxidation. However, ATP is not stored to a great extent in cells, so once muscle contraction starts, more ATP must be made quickly. Since ATP is so important, muscle cells have three different biochemical methods to make it: using creatine phosphate, using glycogen without oxygen, and using aerobic respiration with oxygen, and these methods work together in phases. All these are good until your cells go on strike and refuse to convert the glucose to ATP, then your muscles starve, and your energy comes to a stop.

To put in perspective

Your car broke down and you started running to your appointment. During the first few seconds of running, your muscles are the first to respond to the change in activity level. Your lungs and heart, however, do not react as quickly, and during those beginning steps they do not begin to increase the delivery of oxygen, and the muscles rely on a small amount of ATP that is stored in resting muscles. The stored ATP can provide energy for only a few seconds before it is depleted. Once the stored ATP is just about used up, the body resorts to another high-energy molecule known as creatine phosphate to convert ADP (adenosine diphosphate) to ATP. After about 10 seconds, the stored creatine phosphate in the muscle cells may also be depleted as well.

About 15 seconds into your run, both the stored ATP and creatine phosphate are used up in the muscles. The heart and lungs have still not adapted to the increased need of oxygen. But, no worries, if you haven't made it to your appointment yet, the muscles begin to produce ATP without oxygen by anaerobic metabolism using only glucose obtained from the muscle's own glycogen. A by-product of making ATP without using oxygen is lactic acid. You know when your muscles are building up lactic acid because lactic acid causes tiredness and soreness. It is great that oxygen is not needed, because it takes the heart and lungs some time to get increased oxygen supply to the muscles. Anaerobic metabolism can produce ATP at a rapid pace and will produce enough ATP to last about 90 seconds. But you probably need more ATP than 90 seconds worth to get to your appointment.

You are still not there, but oxygen comes to the rescue, and you keep running. That is because, finally at about 2-3 minutes into your journey, your heart rate and breathing rate have increased to supply more oxygen to your muscles. When oxygen is present, aerobic respiration can take place to break down the glucose for ATP. But at this point, 70-80 percent of the muscle's own glycogen may be depleted, and additional sources are needed. Glucose can then come from several places: remaining glucose supply in the muscle cells, glucose from food in the intestine, glycogen in the liver, fat reserves in the muscles, and in extreme cases (like starvation) the body's protein. Aerobic respiration takes even more chemical reactions to produce ATP than either of the other systems and is the slowest of the three ATP production methods.

Remarkably during exercise your body expedites glucose intake into the cells without the need for aid from insulin! This is because cells have other glucose transport mechanisms that come into play during exercise, the details of which are beyond the scope of this book. During exercise, because muscle cells cannot produce ATP rapidly enough to maintain exercise intensity, insulin is no longer needed to direct glucose delivery to the cells. So, insulin is not required to dock on the insulin receptors to trigger the glucose channels to open. In this situation, the glucose channels open on their own to aid in glucose uptake into the cell without the assistance of insulin, thereby expediting the ATP making process. So, it does not matter if you have insulin resistance, or if you simply do not have enough insulin because when you exercise, your muscles get the glucose they need, and, in turn, your blood glucose level goes down.

Aerobic respiration can supply ATP for several hours or longer, depending on four factors: the total muscle mass, intensity and type of exercise, the level of personal training, and how long the supply of fuel lasts. This is great! But what if your mitochondria are not accepting sugar? If your mitochondria are unhappy and not accepting any work, no amount of sugar albeit "speedy sugar" can make the muscle cells produce the ATP you need. Instead, the unused oxygen and fuel molecules can build up in the cells and cause damage to the cells.

If you get more tired than usual during your run, most likely unbeknownst to you, your cells are not converting the glucose to the ATP you need. You may think you should eat an energy bar or two to give your muscles enough glucose to last for the duration of your journey, but this assumption may not be reality. Although ingesting an energy bar during exercise can attenuate depletion of glycogen, just generating glucose does not necessarily mean the cell will burn it. If your mitochondria are on strike, no amount of glucose you deliver to your cells during your run can talk mitochondria into converting glucose to ATP, unless you satisfy their simple demands: "Do not overload us with incorrect food".

And the saga continues. Despite being tired, you get to your appointment anyway hoping you can rest and recover, but good luck recovering. Remember, unlike during running, when you are at rest, insulin is still needed to direct glucose delivery to the cells to make ATP. In fact, when you are at rest, insulin docks on the insulin receptors and triggers the glucose channels to open. But, again, your cells may not be able to produce the ATP they need for at least two reasons. One, if mitochondria are on strike, they refuse to uptake glucose by blocking the insulin from docking on insulin receptors, thus obstructing opening of the glucose channels. Two, insulin look-a-likes (e.g., lectins from bread), may also play their part in blocking the insulin's receptors. In either case, there is a form of insulin resistance. Sugar-sugar everywhere but you can't use it all, your muscle cells starve, and your energy level drops.

The good news is that it is not too late to prepare for your next exertion. Try satisfying your mitochondria's demands by choosing the correct food within the calories of your ideal weight. So, you keep your mitochondria happy, and they get the glucose they need "for real", to give you the ATP you require for several hours or longer.

Hungry brain

Like muscles, a majority of ATP in the brain is formed in mitochondria. A large portion of ATP energy is used to support neurotransmitters cycling and thus sustaining electrophysiological activity and cell signaling in the brain. The ATP metabolism regulating both ATP production and utilization, plays a fundamental role in cerebral bioenergetics, brain function, and neurodegenerative diseases. No ATP, No signaling.

To better visualize the concept of brain's signaling, think of a wireless phone. The battery must have enough power to send and receive signals, otherwise you may keep saying: "Can you hear me now?". Similarly, the brain must have enough battery power in the form of ATP to communicate signals to and from the rest of your body. Otherwise, your food intake regulation gets interrupted, and you may overeat. Overeating overloads your brain mitochondria. Overloaded brain mitochondria refuse to produce ATP, and a vicious cycle begins.

In the brain, ATP is produced mostly by sugar. As batteries use chemicals to generate power, you eat glucose to provide the sugar needed for generating ATP power, at least you think you do. But not so fast, perception is not reality. Let us think about how normally sugar is delivered to its destination in the brain mitochondria. Insulin first docks on the insulin receptors of the nerve cells or neurons of the brain and signals the glucose channels to open entry for the sugar delivery. Then, sugar gets into the brain in the neurons' mitochondria to generate ATP. However, like the muscles, if your mitochondria are overloaded with work or, for that matter, if your neurons' insulin receptors are blocked by insulin look-a-likes (e.g., lectins from bread), ATP generation comes to a halt. In this situation, the brain can also develop a form of insulin resistance and block entry of sugar at insulin receptors of the neurons. In this case, the neurons insulin receptors are closed for business, the brain neurons get no sugar delivery. Sugar-sugar everywhere but the brain cannot access it, and your brain's energy source, ATP, gets lost or attenuated.

Low ATP in your neurons may also make you overeat by interrupting your food intake regulation. For example, if the hungry brain has little or no reception power, the hungry brain may not receive leptin signals, the stop eating food modulator hormone, to regulate your food intake, and so demands more Calories even if you may be full. Food intake regulation is an important factor involved in the body's weight control. To regulate food intake, the brain must alter your appetite by responding to the hormone signals. But with low ATP power, the hungry brain may resist responding to the hormone signals. The hormones keep asking "Can you hear me now?". Simply put, low ATP power means less messaging, less messaging means less appetite modulation, less appetite modulation means less food regulation, less food regulation means overeating. Overeating means unhappy mitochondria, and unhappy mitochondria means, you guessed it, a less energetic and a more overweight you. The vicious cycle continues.

To empower your brain's communication with the rest of your body, eat correct food in a correct amount to make sure sugar is delivered to the brain mitochondria to create the ATP energy it needs.

8.7 A perfect storm

Let us review what just happened. When mitochondria are exhausted, they do not take it anymore and block entry of sugar into the cells. At the same time, insulin receptors may be blocked by protein look-a-likes which block entry of sugar into the cells as well. So, ATP production comes to a stop, and you get tired. While your energy has come to a stop, more fat is generated at the fat cells, due to additional sugar pumped into the fat cells, instead of being burned in the cells who need it. Concurrently, your fat cells may not release fat to the other cells for oxidation due to too much insulin in your blood.

If this is not a perfect storm, more rain is coming. Simultaneously, because of a lack of ATP, food intake regulation by the brain gets interrupted, and signaling between the appetite modulator hormones (i.e., leptin) and the brain fades. Instead, the brain keeps receiving signals for more food, exhausting your mitochondria even further. The cumulative result leads to many dysfunctions: less muscle mass, hungry brain and nerve cells, sub-optimal heart, liver, and kidney functions, and chubby fat cells. Bear in mind, perception is not reality. Just eating glucose does not mean your cells will get the glucose. Just storing fat does not mean your cells can burn it. And, just eating too much does not mean you get more energy. To get more energy, your body should be in the fat burning state where your mitochondria are happy. To get in the fat burning state, you can simply eat the correct food in a correct amount because there are no magic pills!

8.8 There are no magic pills

Why not take pills to stop overeating and keep mitochondria happy? Why not take hormones to increase appetite-reducing gut hormones and take other hormones to reduce the appetite-stimulant gut hormone ghrelin (hunger hormone). And, while you are at it, why not take supplements or diet products to boost your satiety hormone leptin (the stop-eating hormone) to inhibit appetite stimulation. Yes, you can take supplements/drugs to regulate your food intake through appetite modulation, as some people do, but before you do, you need to know that the process is a little brainy, literally brainy. The hypothalamus is the key region in your brain involved in the regulation of your appetite and thus your weight.

People who use appetite modulators may not have read this book yet. If they did, they would know that for these supplements to work, their mitochondria must be healthy, in the first place, to generate an adequate communication power between the brain and the appetite modulators. As we discussed above, if your mitochondria are not happy enough, they cannot generate adequate power for your brain, so your powerless brain cannot give any marching orders to the appetite modulators. No matter how many supplements you take, they may be wasted along with money for them. But, even if your brain can send marching orders to modulate your appetite, at some point your cells may go on strike and become resistance to the appetite modulators (e.g., leptin resistance). Cells may not accept any more leptin delivery, and appetite regulation may stop. "Resistance is not fun," if you ask insulin.

So, there are no magic pills to take, but here is the good news: there is the Lowellie™ Way. If you use the Lowellie™ Way instead, we believe you may not need to take any supplements or diet products "along with a balanced diet and exercise".

8.9 Take back your power

"I eat a lot, but why am I tired most of the time?" you might ask. For the answer look no further than your question: "I eat a lot," you said! Here is a relevant witty anecdote: someone goes to a doctor and says: "My eye hurts when I drink tea, what should I do?"; "Take the spoon out of your teacup," the doctor says. So, in your case: do not eat a lot.

In other words, to take back your power, stop overeating! Unless, your cells can get a metabolic engine with higher capacity than your current mitochondria, you should not eat a huge number of Calories!! May be hundreds of millions of years from now, new generations of mitochondria will adapt to human overeating and build a bigger engine to handle that ton of spaghetti. But for now, keep your Calories in check and have a balanced diet of correct food and exercise as we suggested in the Lowellie™ Way.

Bear in mind, you are in charge anyway. To control your weight, you have two strategic choices, you can rely on your conscious ability and will power to fight the hunger signal. Or you can stay ahead of the game and decide how much and what you are going to eat ahead of time and win the game without fighting by eating the correct amount of the correct food such as in the Lowellie™ Way. We suggest the latter. If you follow the Lowellie™ Way, we believe you will probably do not have to take leptin or another appetite control supplement, or any supplements as a complement to your diet. Further, you may not need to worry about all the details of brain signaling, biochemistry, etc. The correct amount of the correct food not only provides the energy you need to create more muscle mass, and optimize your brain, heart, kidneys, and liver, it also keeps your fat cells skinny. And above all, the correct amount of the correct food keeps your mitochondria happy. The result could be a more energetic you.

Chapter 9: To Diet or not to Diet, that is the Question!

The human body has been optimized to survive over millions of years and has evolved to give your cells the food fuel they want. Your cells receive the food fuel directly from metabolizing the macronutrients you eat, or from converting one macronutrient to another based-on availability of resources. Rain or shine, your body will try to fuel your cells with an eye on long-term survival, so short-term diet fixes that cut Calories without paying attention to your specific long-term biological requirements may backfire.

Think of your body as a multifuel machine that automatically adjusts the fuel composition and consumption based on feedback from a fuel controller. You choose what food and how much to eat based on feedback from your body processed by your body's controller, your brain. Hunger means you need to eat, appetite tells you what foods taste good, and satiety tells you when you have had enough. The feedback from your body is mostly determined from your genes and your environment, which are specific to you, not like a one-size-fits-all popular diet. Our goal is that you maintain a long-term healthy lifestyle by fueling your body with different types of correct food within the Calories of your ideal weight. So, you can use your body's natural food conversion ability with the correct feedback from your body for your specific biological makeup, and not worry about what diet is popular today.

With your body's natural food conversion ability, your mitochondria can create burnable ATP energy using glucose or ketones as food fuels. The glucose comes from consumed carbs, stored fat, or protein, and the ketones from stored or new fat. If your body has enough available glucose to provide the required energy for your current level of activity, your body uses the glucose to fuel your cells to make ATP. But if there is not enough glucose available, your body begins to break down fat stores and makes glucose from triglycerides or converts amino acids in protein into glucose if needed. If the glucose produced from carbs or stored fat and protein is still insufficient, ketones are used for energy in lieu of glucose, and your liver burns fat to make ketones. If your body steadily burns fat as a fuel source, you lose weight.

Lo and behold, most popular diets also use your body's natural food conversion ability to convert the food resources to food fuel to make ATP. Except, many of them manipulate your available food resources by adjusting how much of each food you should eat, without considering the correct feedback from your body for your specific biological makeup. This may push you into a "yo-yo" of fast weight loss and weight gain. Some may claim, if you want to burn your stored fat, eat less carbs and increase protein. Others may say, if you want to burn even more fat, eat less carbs and decrease your protein. Still others may say, if you want to lose a lot more fat, cut way down on carbs and protein and eat fat! As if your body is their laboratory for experimental diets.

Although these diets may work initially, they may not be a long-term solution to your health, because they may be hard to live with, and may also become undoable overtime. That may be a reason why there are many different low-carb diets that try to improve on the previous ones. One of the latest is a low-carb, low-protein, high-fat ketogenetic diet. We will help you navigate some of the ins and outs of low-carb diets over the next couple of sections, as well as their possible benefits and drawbacks. Once you know how food works behind the scenes to fuel your cells, and how these diets may or may not work for you, you can determine which food or diet is for you or not and why. Or you may ultimately choose a balanced diet of correct food within the Calories of your ideal weight to include all types of foods that you like—as we do.

9.1 Low-carb diets

Carbohydrates may be the tiniest fraction of you, but they end up creating almost all the ATP energy. Low-carb diets are generally designed to burn fat at higher rates by keeping your carbohydrate intake lower than about 50 grams per day. In this manner, when your body requires additional energy, these diets intend to encourage your body to enter and stay in a state called ketosis. Ketosis refers to the metabolic state in which the body converts fat into ketones. The low-carb-diets generally rely on ketosis and use your body's natural food conversion ability to try to encourage ketosis one way or another. But this is where most of them fail, in sustaining ketosis!

We will explain the sustaining ketosis caveat in the next section. But first, let's look at how your body can achieve ketosis in the first place. Regardless of what diet you are on, your body naturally follows the path of least resistance. Your body goes to burning glucose first, because it is easier and more efficient than burning fat. If your blood sugar levels are too high, your body regulates glucose by the pancreas signaling the liver to convert excess glucose to glycogen to store it for later use. To achieve ketosis and start burning fat, you need to use up both glucose and glycogen first.

You can use up glucose by minimizing carbs, but once you burn up the glucose, glycogen is next in line to fuel your cells when needed. Glycogen is one of the reasons why you do not need to eat every fifteen to twenty minutes. Your body typically has blood glucose levels that can sustain all cellular processes for three to four hours. If you do not eat in that time frame, your body will begin to break down the glycogen it has stored to keep your body running. But glycogen supplies are limited, and you will run out of glycogen too. Then what? You enter ketosis and start burning existing fat and producing ketones. So, ketosis is a primary premise of low-carb diets if you can sustain it.

But sustaining ketosis may be a challenge unless you are trapped in a cave. Imagine you are trapped in a cave in Thailand, you have not eaten for a week, a volcano erupted outside, and the corner pizza does not deliver. Then, ketosis sends the food rescue team ketones, to feed you until the escape pod arrives. While you are waiting for the escape pod to rescue you from the cave, your body can sustain ketosis and make ketones as a dominant food fuel by burning your existing body fat already stored in your fat cells, so you lose weight.

However, there is no profit without a risk. Like the "trapped in a cave" example above, ketones can be increased during fasting, starving, low-carb diets, prolonged exercise, and untreated type 1 diabetes mellitus. In these situations, you can sustain ketosis for a while, but there is a price to pay for not consuming enough carbs, you may lose muscle mass. This is because, on a low-carb diet although most of the brain can use ketones, there are portions that require glucose to function. When carbs are eliminated or minimized, ketones can only provide up to 70% of the brain's energy needs, the other 30% needing glucose. In this circumstance, at least for the first few days of carbs restriction, protein in your muscles is converted to "new" glucose in a process called gluconeogenesis to rescue your brain at the expense of reducing muscle mass. Without continual replenishment, your muscles like the rest of your body will be reduced through normal attrition. Luckily, because your body wants to preserve energy and muscle mass, the body changes strategy and tries to use ketosis to produce ketones again, subject to the sustainability caveat as we will discuss below.

Low-carb diets' caveat

The premise of losing weight on a low-carb diet, whether high protein or high fat, is plausible with one caveat: are you consuming ketones by staying in a state of ketosis? Half as much effort is needed to turn ketones into ATP as turning glucose into ATP, so ketones are mitochondria's favorite fuel especially during slow burn such as at night. At night when you are not eating, mitochondria slow down and use ketones to create ATP, which also means you are burning fat making the ketones and losing weight.

You might ask, if mitochondria are so happy with burning ketones, why not burn fat to make ketones all the time and lose weight while you are at it? Because, for your wish to be granted, you must stay in a state of ketosis, which is a state that is not easily sustainable. To stay in ketosis your insulin level must be low. For your insulin level to be low, you should have a low sugar level in your blood, and to have a low sugar level, you should keep both your carbs and protein low enough. But as we will explain below, most likely in, for example a low-carb high-protein diet, both carbs and protein team-up to spike the sugar causing an increase in your insulin level in response, negating ketosis.

So, why does a high insulin level block ketosis? Because your mitochondria cannot process fat directly from your fat cells so your stored fat must first be turned into ketones, indirectly, by the enzyme hormone-sensitive lipase (HSL). But, as we previously explained, insulin is the main hormone to which HSL is sensitive and, remarkably enough, your brain has its priorities straight. Before HSL turns any fat to ketones, your brain senses your insulin level first to check if you are protecting yourself from an upcoming food shortage! If your insulin level is high, your brain gets a signal that you are eating for an upcoming food shortage. Your brain then directs conversion of available food into fat for a rainy day and assumes the last thing you want to do is to convert fat to ketones. In this manner, the high insulin level keeps HSL from doing its job of making ketones for your mitochondria, thus blocking ketosis.

Moreover, because your body is very protective of you, excess insulin does not stop there, it goes all out to make new fat. Excess insulin activates the enzyme lipoprotein lipase (LPL) to use any leftover glucose, beyond what the liver can hold as glycogen, for conversion to fat. To make the situation worse, if you have been eating too much and have overworked your mitochondria, they will stop accepting any more work by resisting insulin. And if you recall from Chapter 7, insulin does not take resistance lightly and in response instructs the enzyme LPL to make fat cells turn sugar into more fat for storage. So, if your insulin level is high, you not only don't burn old fat to make ketones, but you also add new fat.

Thereby, many low-carb diets fail. They disregard the possibility of excess insulin in your blood. They count on you to keep the carbs very low by not eating too much protein, and have an exceptionally low-carb diet, so you keep your insulin level low unblocking HSL to turn fat into ketone, thus maintaining ketosis. Good luck keeping the carbs that low, unless you are trapped in a cave.

So, if you are on a high-protein low-carb diet and you are not losing weight and wondering why, you may ask yourself: "I am eating a lot of protein and only a few carbs, so why am I not losing fat?". The answer lies in your question itself. You may be eating only a few carbs to keep the glucose low, but do not forget, you said you are also eating "a lot of protein", which can also convert to glucose. Those extra carbs can result in your carbs being higher than 50 grams, and thus may block stored fat from turning into ketones. This is a dilemma that may occur with high-protein, low-carb diets. Followers of these diets may think they are eating few carbs, but, unbeknownst to them, they add a lot of carbs by eating extra protein that may be converted to carbs. Thereby, they do not get ketones. Instead, they get a headache, low energy, and keep the fat.

These low-carb diets may work, if you stay in ketosis all the time, which requires really keeping the carbs low, and thus keeping the insulin level low. This raises a good question. Since high protein may cause high carbs and thus a high insulin level, what if you eat less protein to stay in ketosis? There you go again, here comes yet another diet. A century old, low-carb, low-protein, high-fat Ketogenic diet, resurfaced as a new popular "Keto" diet to encourage ketosis.

Ketogenic diet

The ketogenic diet focuses on burning fat to produce ketones. In diet discussions, ketones and ketone bodies are used interchangeably, but they are not the same thing. There are millions of ketone compounds that are naturally occurring with different chemical structures, but not all of them are ketone bodies. The term ketones in diet discussions refers to ketone bodies which are a type of water-soluble subset of ketones that your body forms naturally from metabolizing fatty acids. There are three ketones that your body produces: acetoacetate, beta-hydroxybutyrate (BHB), and acetone, as such they fall under the category of "ketone bodies". Thus, all ketone bodies are ketones, but not all ketones are ketone bodies. For example, since acetone is both naturally occurring and produced by your body it is simultaneously a ketone and a ketone body. An example of a non-ketone-body ketone is Diacetyl, which is used to give buttery flavor to candy, popcorn, and baked goods.

The ketogenic diet or Keto diet has its roots in the century old therapeutic ketogenic diet. Keto diets are low-carb, low-protein, high-fat diets that are designed to make you burn fat as your main source of energy. The key to a Keto diet is eating fat that does not make your insulin level go up, as eating carbs or protein would. In other words, a purpose of the Keto diet is to prevent spikes in your insulin level, so you do not store fat. Instead, you burn the fat, creating the ketones that give you an effective and efficient metabolic jolt. The high-fat Keto diet is also a form of extremely low-carb diet. A significant difference between a Keto diet and most other low-carb diets is that the Keto diet reduces protein significantly and relies on burning fat.

Most of the time, your body burns sugar from carbohydrates and protein for energy, but if you cut off your body's supply of carbs and protein, your body begins seeking out fat instead. Reducing carbs and protein and eating fat instead may shift you into a state of ketosis, the state in which you stop using sugar for the most part and start using ketones as the dominant food fuel required by ketosis. Keto diets are designed to increase your chances of entering and staying in the state of ketosis compared to low-carb, high-protein diets. In Keto diets, with about 5-10% carbohydrates, 10-20% protein, and 70-80% fat for your total daily Calories, your body is supposed to enter ketosis, and start burning fat as its main source of fuel.

Yes, if you keep your carbohydrate intake low, and do not eat too much protein, you may reap the benefits of staying in ketosis and burning fat for fuel. But on the con side, like other low-carb diets, most people on Keto diets do not enter, or stay in ketosis, because they do not keep the protein, "the hidden carb", as low as they should. Keto gives you ketosis, only if you can keep it.

Also, a common misconception in Keto is that you burn stored body fat all the time. Make no mistake, just because you are using fat as your main ATP source, it does not mean you are constantly burning through your stored body fat. You will use the fat you eat first, and the stored body fat after that. So, unlike most low-carb, high-protein diets, you will not be burning stored body fat all the time in Keto.

Furthermore, some followers of Keto say mainly two "good things" about Keto: you may be able to burn body fat without feeling hungry all the time, and may burn about 300 more Calories per day than their higher-carb counterparts. But these "good things" are not unique to Keto. If you remember from Chapter 7, protein and oxygen are also fat burners, so they can serve the same purpose as these "good things" without the challenges associated with ketosis. Protein suppresses appetite, so like Keto you may as well be able to burn body fat without feeling hungry all the time and may burn more Calories per day if you incorporate high protein in your diet. Plus, you can burn even more Calories than Keto by breathing more oxygen through exercising more. After all, the low-protein idea in Keto may not help you stay in ketosis anyway. So, why not have a balanced diet of correct food with higher protein, and exercise regularly, instead of being on Keto where the emperor has no clothes, where the Keto has no ketosis.

However, despite challenges associated with ketosis, on the pro side, Keto diets may have some benefits regarding a variety of diseases. Keto diets may help people with diabetes and their insulin level. Keto diets can also be used to treat clinical conditions, primarily epilepsy. Literature on the subject also suggest possible benefits for other brain conditions such as Parkinson's and Alzheimer's diseases. So, the brain is happily deriving energy from ketones, sure, but why would this be protective against such a variety of brain diseases? One answer may be energy. Despite their superficial differences, many neurological diseases share one major problem, deficient energy production. During metabolic stress, ketones serve as an alternative energy source to maintain normal brain cell metabolism.

But "No risk No glory", although ketones can be beneficial to brain functions, they are not always neuroprotective. Sometimes they can be toxic for the brain (e.g., the ketone acetone can be used as nail polish remover). Ketones may also be related to a dangerous diabetic complication called ketoacidosis resulting from dangerously high levels of ketones and blood sugar, which can occur if insulin levels are far too low. As an example, ketoacidosis is a dangerous complication of diabetes mellitus or alcoholism. In extreme cases of ketoacidosis, high concentrations of ketones may alter the acid/alkaline balance (pH balance) of blood and may tip a person into a coma.

So, what should be the next new popular diet? A balanced diet of correct food and exercise!?:)

9.2 So, diet or not diet?

Before we answer this question, let's recap some of the pros and cons of low-carb diets briefly.

On the pro side, most low-carb diets encourage ketosis, so your body can burn fat at a high enough rate, to produce a lot of ketones. These ketones are favorable food fuel for your cells and may alone provide enough energy for the parts of the body that cannot metabolize fatty acids such as part of the brain. This may be the reason that ketosis is used to treat clinical conditions related to the brain.

On the con side, even though ketones are favorable for most cells, especially brain cells, some tissues still require at least some glucose, which is not normally made from fat. In a very low-carb diet, glucose can be made in the liver and kidneys using protein from

127

elsewhere in the body. OO! But take care, if not enough protein is provided by the diet as in Keto, the body starts chewing on muscle cells. But wait a minute, if there is excess protein as in low-carb, high-protein diets, then the protein converts into too much glucose, and the excess glucose turns on the insulin's fountain that stops fat burning, and thus ketone production. Even if you make ketones, an overly high amount of them may be toxic to your brain and/or cause dangerous diabetic complications anyway. Finally, in a low-carb, high-fat diet such as Keto you burn the new fat first instead of burning your existing body fat, giving your waistline a pass.

But the good news is that you do not necessarily have to take the risk associated with the cons to profit from the pros. Because ketones are not unusual food fuels for your body, they don't start and end with low-carb diets. As such, they are always present in your blood, albeit not always as a dominant food fuel as required by ketosis. For example, ketones are produced in small amounts whenever you go for many hours without eating such as during a full night's sleep. In fact, your heart and the ultrafiltration part of the kidneys (i.e., renal cortex) are using ketones as fuel right now because these cells prefer to use ketones instead of sugar anyway.

Even if you would like to add more ketones to your diet than your body naturally makes, you do not need low-carb-diets such as Keto, you can just eat them! Get them from good sources of fat instead such as medium-chain triglycerides (MCT) oil, coconut oil, palm kernel oil, and from increasing time between meals. Although these ketone boosting fats aren't ketones themselves, they can be broken down into ketones in the liver whether the body is in ketosis or not. And as for being in ketosis to lose fat, most people can lose fat and make ketones without being in ketosis anyway. If you have a balanced diet of correct food within the Calories of your ideal weight, you can burn the extra fat gradually through time. In other words, if you create a calorie deficit, you can burn fat even if you are not in ketosis. So, if you eat slightly less than your body needs, your body must gain energy from somewhere else, such as the fat in your waistline.

In summation, although there may be some benefits in some part of one diet or another, they are not as simple as a balanced diet and exercise.

To this end, our answer to this conundrum of "diet or not diet?" is "not fad diets". Instead, we choose a balanced diet and exercise as we described in the *Lowellie™ Way*. In this *"Way"*, you most likely do not create excess carbs to create excess insulin, and your body will lose the extra fat through time if you stay in Calorie deficit. Lo and behold, in the process, ketones are made in moderation in your liver from fatty acids found in your food, or your own body fat, and are used for energy in lieu of carbs. As your body steadily burns fat as food fuel, you will start to lose weight without entering extreme ketosis. So, if you are healthy, there is no need to enter non-sustainable extreme ketosis, encouraged by some popular low-carb diets, to lose weight.

As we mentioned above, the "along with a balanced diet and exercise" is the title of our book, because, if you have a balanced diet and exercise, you may get good results regardless of products and fad diets foisted on you. We suggest you skip fad diets and just go straight to the *Lowellie™ Way*. Why not, have a balanced diet of correct food with a proper quantity of macronutrients within the Calories of your ideal weight. So, burn your already stored body fat to lose weight, and as a bonus, keep your muscle mass too. You could do that instead of wasting your time burning new fat that you just added in a diet such as Keto. Why, the risk with no glory? Skip being worried about whether entering ketosis, or not, or whether your body produces dangerously high levels of ketones associated with ketosis, or not. And most deliciously, eat what you like in correct amounts.

Use the information we provide in this book to create a well-informed personalized balanced diet for life with the Lowellie™ Way. Instead of engaging in the next popular diet that would last only a few weeks to months, try to embrace change that is sustainable over the long term. A balanced diet from the correct food such as very colorful fruits and vegetables, meat, dairy products, nuts, and legumes in a correct amount, and regular exercise seems to have the best evidence for a long healthier vibrant life. So, you are all set, no need for extreme measures.

Chapter 10: Basic Macronutrients and Their Ratio

Most people know the basic macronutrients that a person needs are carbohydrates, fats, and proteins. But we find it interesting that most people may not know the fundamentals of these macronutrients such as what they are made of, what they do, and how much of each is needed. Well informed choices of what to eat, how much to eat, and in what ratio, lead to an independent long-term healthy lifestyle. A lifestyle free of endless diets and the diet products advertised daily.

Because your body is energy efficient, if all three macronutrients are abundant in your diet, carbohydrates and fats will be used primarily for energy, while proteins provide the raw materials for making hormones, muscle, and other essential biological parts. Alternatively, when glucose is in short supply, ketones are made in lieu of carbohydrates in the liver from the breakdown of fats. Ketone production mostly occurs overnight, and during dieting or fasting. Carbohydrates, ketones, and proteins provide approximately 4 Calories (17 kilo Joule) of energy per gram, and fats provide approximately 9 Calories (37 kilo Joule) per gram. To keep a healthy lifestyle, it is important to keep a healthy ratio of these macronutrients so you can stay within the Calories of your target weight.

10.1 Protein: The largest fraction of you without which life would not be possible

If carbohydrates provide energy, and fats insulate and store energy, then just about everything else is done by proteins. They form the bulk of your muscles and connective tissues, but they are also what the ion channels and pumps (e.g., glucose channels) in cell walls of your neurons and muscle cells are made of. Proteins also make up your enzymes which are a type of specialized protein molecules in your cells that work as biological catalysts, and which are responsible for most of the chemical reactions in your body. In other words, your body runs on protein and pretty much is protein.

For example, many chemical reactions are catalyzed by enzymes, where an increase in reaction rate caused by enzymatic catalysis can be 17 orders of magnitude over an uncatalyzed reaction. So, some reactions that would take millions of years without an enzyme could take only milliseconds with the enzyme! How long do you think it would take to breakdown glucose to make ATP to run your body without the enzymes? Yes, you guessed right, perhaps millions of years. So, without protein, life would not be possible.

Proteins are building blocks for your biological parts. Protein is a large structural molecule with one or more molecular chains assembled out of basic units called amino acids, many of which the body cannot produce on its own. The elements of an amino acid are carbon, hydrogen, oxygen, and nitrogen. After you eat protein-containing foods, they are digested and broken down into individual amino acids which cells then use to rebuild new proteins. Those amino acids then get reassembled using anabolic reactions into your very own proteins as defined by your DNA.

Many foods do not provide every essential amino acid, but when you eat meat or animal products (e.g., fish, and eggs) you generally do get all the essential amino acids. This is important because, after water, you are mostly made of protein, on the order of sixteen percent of your body. You do not have to eat animal products to get the protein you need, although they are the highest protein and lowest carb nutrition sources. But if you do not eat animal products, you may need to be more creative to get the same essential amino acids from plant-based foods. You may have to eat more carbs to achieve the same amount of protein from vegetables as from comparable animal products.

At any rate, you can eat protein from whatever high-protein correct food sources you prefer such as meats, dairy products, eggs, legumes, and nuts. Glutamine protein found, for example, in animal products, can also be found in beans or cabbage, and may improve intestine function and aid the immune system. The amino acid cysteine is readily available in many correct foods such as whey, broccoli, brussels sprouts, egg yolks, garlic, onions, and poultry. Cysteine may improve functioning of the immune system, chronic respiratory conditions, fertility, and brain health.

Because almost everything you eat was once alive and every cell of every living thing contains protein, if you are eating the correct foods, you are at least partially restocking your protein supplies. So, how much of your Calorie intake should be allocated to protein?

How much protein do you need?

A daily dietary reference intake (DRI) from available literature for protein is 10-35% of your daily Caloric intake. For example, the DRI for protein is 0.36 grams per pound of body weight (0.8 grams per kilogram) which is only about 46 grams per day for the average woman, and 56 grams per day for the average man. If you weigh 175 pounds (79 kilograms) and your daily Caloric intake is 2,275 Calories, you need about 63 grams of protein per day, which is about 11% of your daily Calorie intake. This amount of protein intake may be enough to prevent deficiency to stay healthy but may be far from optimal if you are trying to improve your general health, lose weight, or gain muscle. Higher amounts of protein intake may be recommended for various health goals.

If you are at a healthy weight, do not lift weights, and do not exercise much, then aiming for 0.36 to 0.6 grams of protein per pound (0.8 to 1.3 grams per kilogram) of body weight may be a reasonable estimate. This amounts to 63-105 grams of protein per day if you weigh 175 pounds, which comprises an 11%-18% protein intake, if your daily Caloric intake is 2,275 Calories. A protein intake at around 15%, or about 85 grams may be optimal for looking to be generally healthy.

To lose weight, aiming for 25-35% of Calories as protein may be optimal. Using the same example as above, if you weigh 175 pounds (79 kilograms) and your daily Caloric intake is 2,275 Calories, then a 30% protein intake is 170 grams, which is about 1 gram per pound of body weight. A protein intake range of around 25%-30%, or 142-170 grams for this example, may also be optimal for gaining muscles.

Calculators on the Internet can give you a broad range for acceptable daily protein intake. You can also multiply your weight in pounds by the grams of protein you think you need per pound of your body weight (e.g., 0.36 to 1 gram). Alternatively, you can calculate your recommended daily protein intake in grams customized to your daily Caloric needs as follows: multiply your daily Caloric needs by a percent of Calories that you think you need from protein (e.g., 0.3 for 30%), then divide by 4 (number of Calories per gram of protein).

For example, you can find the number of grams you would eat for 30% protein intake by multiplying your daily Calorie intake by 0.3 and divide it by 4, or simply multiply your daily Calorie intake by 0.075 (which is 0.3 divided by 4). As in the above example, if you weigh 175 pounds (79 kilograms) and are on a 2,275 Calorie diet, you should eat (2,275 * 0.075) = 170 grams of protein per day for weight loss. That would be equivalent to about 29 oz of skinless chicken breast or salmon, or 68 oz of lentils per day. It may be best to spread your protein intake throughout the day by eating protein with every meal for 3-5 meals a day (or 8 meals if you are a Hobbit).

Variations of protein intake

Since human protein intake varies, many variations of protein intake may be recommended. Keep in mind that these recommended numbers may not need to be exact, anything in your chosen range (e.g., 25-35% of Caloric intake) for protein intake may be effective for your health goal depending on how you synthesize protein.

Protein synthesis is an important factor in how much protein you may need. There are factors that decrease protein synthesis and make your muscles less sensitive to protein signaling thus increasing your need for protein. Getting older and/or being inactive is one of them, which is a reason why older adults seem to need up to 50% higher than DRI (e.g., about 0.45 to 0.6 grams of protein per pound of body weight per day, rather than 0.36 grams) to max out their rates of protein synthesis. This may help prevent osteoporosis and muscle mass reduction. You may wish to check with your doctor. People who are recovering from injuries may also need more protein. But is it really age that causes this "anabolic resistance", or is it simply a consequence of an unfortunate habit of becoming less physically active as we age?

The good news is that you can increase protein synthesis by increasing muscle-signaling capacity. The following two routines can provide a good way to increase muscle-signaling capacity: exercise before you eat so your muscles become more sensitive to protein's signals, and just eat the protein before you go to sleep, a pre-bedtime dose of protein may boost muscle synthesis as you sleep.

Too much of a good thing may not be so good

Since there may be significant benefits, it may be better for most people to err on the side of more protein rather than less. However, because too much of a good thing may not be so good, you should be aware of how much protein is generally considered safe, tolerable, or may cause health issues. Long-term consumption of protein at 2 grams per kilogram body weight per day is generally considered safe for healthy adults, and the tolerable upper limit is generally considered to be 3.5g per kilogram (per 2.2 pounds) body weight per day for some well-adapted subjects such as athletes. Chronic high protein intake (>2g per kilogram body weight per day for adults) may result in digestive, renal, and vascular abnormalities and should usually be avoided. So, if you are 175 pounds (79 kilograms), 160 grams per day may be okay.

10.2 Fat: The sixteen percent of you—some of which you may want to get rid of

Fat is a fuel for generating ATP in your cells' mitochondria. Fat typically provides more than half of the body's energy needs and enables the transport of fat-soluble vitamins. Fat further helps maintain cell function, insulates you and protects your vital organs, helps proteins do their jobs, and contributes to flavor and texture. After all, fat cells are like gas stations of your body. If you have used up all your available glucose from other sources such as carbohydrates and proteins, then cells get their fuel from the fat cells to create ATP. And that can be how you lose fat!

Just like carbohydrates, molecules of fat comprise carbon, hydrogen, and oxygen atoms. Triglycerides are a main form of fat in foods and are a major stored form of fat in the body. Triglycerides are comprised of long chains of glycerol molecules, each of which is attached to three (tri) molecules of fatty acids, hence the name "triglyceride". Fatty acids that are not needed right away are repackaged into triglyceride bundles and stored in fat cells which have a large capacity for providing fuel for your cells when they need them. People are very good at storing fat.

Triglycerides are linked together in specific patterns. It is the different combinations of these atoms that create most of the difference in types of fats. Fats may be classified as unsaturated fats ("Good" fats), saturated fats ("Not-So-Bad" fats), and trans fats ("Bad" fats), depending on the detailed structure of the fatty acids involved.

"Good" fats

Among its many attributes, "Good" fats or unsaturated fats maintain normal nerve and brain impulses, may help prevent arthritis, and may be used to treat or prevent psoriasis and eczema. Unsaturated fats are also necessary for normal brain development, help produce new body cells, and are necessary for prostaglandin production, and healthy skin and hair. And perhaps among the most popular functions of unsaturated fat is their ability to lower risk of cardiovascular diseases (CVDs) by reducing risk of blood clots, decreasing blood pressure, and decreasing low density lipoproteins (bad cholesterol LDL). Unsaturated fats are also known to decrease very low-density cholesterol (another bad cholesterol, VLDL) and triglyceride levels, and increase high-density lipoproteins (good cholesterol, HDL).

A quick note on triglyceride levels. As we mentioned previously, your fat is primarily made of triglycerides. So why should you be concerned with triglyceride levels? The issue is generally the triglyceride level in your blood because a high triglyceride level may indicate that triglycerides and other fats may be moving via your blood to places they should not be. For example, a high triglyceride level may indicate fat is building up in your arteries causing a risk of stroke, and heart attack.

Unsaturated fats may lower the risk of disease because they are most likely liquid at room temperature and as such generally do not block your arteries. Here is a little science behind it. What makes them unsaturated is their carbon–carbon double bonds in their molecular structure. The more double bonds, the more bending in their carbon chain, and the more bending makes them hard to pack in density. Imagine packing straws in a tube vs. packing coils in a tube, the coils are harder to pack in a dense configuration than straws. The harder they are to pack, the more likely they are to be liquid at room temperature. So, if you have many of these carbon–

carbon double bonds as in polyunsaturated fat, the carbon chain is very bendy and even more likely be liquid at room temperature. Being liquid at room temperature may mean they are less likely to be solid in your arteries and your blood vessels and may provide a lower risk of disease.

The good news is that, when you are choosing fat, you do not really need to look where and how much their carbon chains are curved (not that you could tell with your eyes anyway). Instead, you can choose correct foods high in unsaturated fats as we discuss in Chapter 12.

"Not-So-Bad" fats

While not as harmful as trans fats, by comparison with unsaturated fats, "Not-So-Bad" fats or saturated fats negatively impact health and are best consumed in moderation. Compared to unsaturated fat, saturated fats have a carbon chain with no carbon-carbon double bound in their fatty acid chains and are "saturated" because they have their maximum of hydrogen atoms on the carbon atoms. With no carbon-carbon double bounds there is little or no bending in the carbon chain, which makes saturated fat easy to densely pack like packing straws in a tube and likely to be solid at room temperature. Saturated fats such as butter and lard are usually solid at room temperature and may thus be stickier in your blood stream. Saturated fats are typically fats from animal products, though some oils such as palm and coconut have saturated fats too. Avoid or minimize foods containing large amounts of saturated fats such as beef, butter, cheese, and ice cream.

"Bad" fats

"Bad" fats or trans fats increase disease risk, even when eaten in small quantities. Foods containing trans fats are primarily highly processed foods made with trans fats such as partially hydrogenated oil. Trans fats have their hydrogen atoms in a "trans configuration" that is not typically found in nature, that causes the carbon chain to remain straight without bends and are easily densely packed like packing straws in a tube. Thus, the chemical structure is more likely to be solid like margarine.

Trans fats are rare in nature and foods from natural sources and are typically created in an industrial process called (partial) hydrogenation. Trans fats have possible negative health effects such as increased risk of bad cholesterol blood levels, atherosclerosis, cardiovascular diseases (CVDs), obesity, type 2 diabetes, insulin resistance, and certain cancers and chronic disorders.

So, avoid fats with no bends in their molecular structure! Or simply avoid high trans-fat foods such as margarine, fried foods, and highly processed foods. Fortunately, trans fats have been eliminated from many foods by the food industry.

10.3 How much fat do you need?

The daily dietary reference intake (DRI) for fat in adults is 20% to 35% of total Caloric needs from fat. That is about 50-88 grams of fat per day if you eat 2,275 Calories per day. Like protein, calculators on the Internet can give you a broad range for acceptable fat intake. Alternatively, you can calculate your recommended fat intake customized to your daily needs as follows: multiply your daily Caloric needs by a percent of Calories that you think you need from fat (e.g., 0.2 for 20%), then divide by 9 (number of Calories per gram of fat). Or simply, multiply your daily Calorie intake by 0.022 (which is 0.2 divided by 9). If you weigh 175 pounds (79 kilograms) and are on a 2,275 Calorie diet, you will need 2,275 * 0.022 = 50 grams of fat per day.

Here is a list to give you an idea about fat content of some example foods: 8.9 grams in 1 oz (28g) of dark chocolate, 20 grams in one classic plain cake donut, 10 grams in a small slice of apple pie, 2 grams in 1 oz (28g) or about 18 potato chips, 14 grams in 1 oz (28g) or about 24 almonds, 2.14 grams in 1 oz (28g) skinless salmon, 1 gram in 1 oz (28g) skinless chicken, 12 grams in 1/2 medium avocado, 5 grams in 1 oz (28g) steak, 5 grams in 1 egg, 0.5 grams in 1 oz (28g) ham, 0 grams in egg whites, and 14 grams in 1 tablespoon of olive oil. We like potato chips, pie, and donuts but we have them only as a treat occasionally because they are high in saturated fat and highly processed unless we make them at home.

Here is the thing, you may from time to time overdue your fat intake for one of your meals, that is, you may have a large piece of pizza or a big steak for lunch, but no worries, try to compensate for it by having a zero-fat dinner. For example, you may have a zero-fat dinner such as kale-lentil soup, shrimps with steamed vegetables, mushroom soup with vegetable broth or bone broth, or a zero-fat smoothie with kale and liquid egg white.

10.4 Carbohydrates: The tiniest fraction of you, "the troublemaker that you love"

Only about one percent of you is carbohydrates (carbs). "Carbo" means carbon, while "hydrate" means water or its elements. But like fat, carbohydrate molecules really mean a combination of carbon, hydrogen, and oxygen atoms, which have energy levels close to the fuel for your car. In fact, some carbohydrate foods such as corn are converted into fuel for cars (e.g., ethanol, and biodiesel).

Carbohydrates are "the troublemaker that you love" that feels so good when you eat it but not so good when you go on the weight scale. Glucose is a carbohydrate that is your primary source of energy and is critical for the normal function of most cells. To get glucose, your body first goes to carbs and then to protein and fat. Carbohydrates may be classified into two main types: simple including monosaccharides and disaccharides often called "sugars" or "simple sugars", and complex including polysaccharides.

Monosaccharides such as glucose, fructose (in fruits), and galactose contain one sugar unit. Glucose and fructose are found in fruits and vegetables, as well as honey, corn syrup, and high fructose corn syrup. Fructose is special because it is the sweetest carbohydrate. Plants make a lot of fructose as a way of attracting insects and animals, which help plants to reproduce. Galactose is found in milk and dairy products made from milk, but it is almost always linked to glucose to form a disaccharide (lactose). You rarely find Galactose in your food supply in monosaccharide form.

Disaccharides contain two sugar units. There are three naturally occurring disaccharides in human nutrition: maltose (glucose bonded to glucose), sucrose (glucose bonded to fructose), and lactose (glucose bonded to galactose).

Maltose is made of two glucose molecules bonded together. It doesn't occur naturally in any appreciable amount in foods, with one exception sprouted grains. Grains contain a lot of starch, which is made of long chains of glucose, and when the seed of a grain starts to sprout, it begins to break down that starch, creating maltose. If bread is made from those sprouted grains, that bread will have some maltose. Sprouted grain bread is usually a little heavier and sweeter than bread made from regular flour. Maltose also plays a role in the production of beer and liquor because this process involves the fermentation of grains or other carbohydrate sources. Maltose is formed during the breakdown of those carbohydrates but there is very little remaining once the fermentation process is complete. You can taste the sweetness of maltose if you hold a starchy food in your mouth for a minute or so. Try this with a simple food like a cracker. Starch is not sweet, but as the starch in the cracker is broken down by enzymes in your saliva, maltose will form, and you'll taste the sweetness!

Sucrose is made of a glucose molecule bonded to a fructose molecule. It is made by plants for the same reason as fructose, to attract animals to eat the fruit or vegetable containing sucrose and spread seeds. Sucrose is naturally occurring in fruits and vegetables, and most fruits and vegetables contain a mixture of glucose, fructose, and sucrose. Sucrose is also found in maple syrup and honey.

Humans have figured out how to concentrate sugars such as sucrose and fructose in plants such as sugar cane, sugar beets, and corn to make refined products like table sugar and corn syrup. The sucrose and fructose found in a sweet potato is chemically identical to the sucrose found in table sugar and corn syrup. But here is the thing, what is different is the package the sugars come in. When you eat a sweet potato or a fig, you also get lots of fiber, vitamins, and minerals in that package, whereas sugar and corn syrup only provide sugar, nothing else. However, you don't have to eat sugar to get glucose, but if you like sugar, pay attention to the package it comes in, and how much of it you eat to keep your insulin in check.

Lactose is made of a glucose molecule bonded to a galactose molecule. It is sometimes called "milk sugar" as it is found in dairy products such as milk, yogurt, and cheese. These are some of the few animal foods that have high amounts of carbohydrates. Most of our carbohydrates come from plant foods.

Polysaccharides or complex polysaccharides such as starch, glycogen and fiber contain three or more sugar units. They are often referred to as "complex" carbohydrates because they are typically long multiple-branched chains of sugar units. These are basically many simple sugars linked together.

Starch is the storage form of carbohydrates in plants. Plants make starch to store glucose. For example, starch is in seeds to give the seedling energy to sprout, and we eat those seeds in the form of seeds, grains, nuts, and legumes such as soybeans, lentils, pinto beans, and kidney beans. Starch is also stored in roots and tubers to provide stored energy for the plant to grow and reproduce, and people eat these in the form of potatoes, sweet potatoes, carrots, beets, and turnips.

When you eat plant foods with starch, you can break it down into glucose to provide fuel for your body's cells. In addition, starch from whole plant foods comes packaged with other valuable nutrients. Also refined starch such as corn starch is an ingredient in many highly processed foods, because it serves as a good thickener.

Glycogen is the storage form of carbohydrates in animals, humans included. It is made up of highly branched chains of glucose, and it is stored in the liver and skeletal muscles. The branched structure of glycogen makes it easier to break down quickly to release glucose to serve as fuel when needed on short notice. Liver glycogen is broken down into glucose, which is released into the bloodstream and can be used by cells around the body. Muscle glycogen provides energy usually only for muscle to fuel activity. That can come in handy if you are being chased by a tiger or running to make your train! Even though glycogen is stored in the liver and muscles of animals, we do not find it in meat, because it breaks down soon after slaughter. Thus, glycogen is not found in our food. Instead, we must make it in our liver and muscle from glucose.

Complex carbs take longer to digest and absorb since their sugar units must be separated into their monosaccharides before absorption. For this reason, most "complex" carbohydrates are called "good carbs". In contrast, simple carbohydrates are absorbed quickly, and therefore raise blood-sugar levels more rapidly than other nutrients. Spikes in blood glucose levels after ingestion of simple sugars may be related to some heart and vascular diseases. So, if you like carbs, maximize the complex ones and minimize the simple ones.

The main thing you need to know is that glucose is the be-all end-all molecular fuel that most of your cells need to make ATP. Your cells use ATP to drive anabolic reactions when they need to make new polymers or get anything else done. Now some of your cells can get their energy from fats and protein, but many of the most important ones, like your neurons and red blood cells, feed exclusively on glucose. That is why most of the carbs that you eat are converted to glucose. But rest assured, if you don't like carbs or want to reduce weight by cutting back on your carbs, fat and protein gets converted to glucose too. Your cells get the glucose they need one way or the other.

Carbohydrate-rich foods can cause carbohydrate addiction

Carbohydrate addiction is a compelling hunger, craving, or desire for carbohydrate-rich foods, and can result in a growing hunger for starches, snack foods, junk food, and sweets. Here comes insulin again, the fat saver. Carbohydrate addiction is caused by an over release of the hormone insulin when carbohydrate-rich foods are eaten. Elevations in insulin produce increased hunger and heighten perceived pleasantness of sweet taste. Insulin functions as a hunger hormone that signals your body to take in food. Once the food is consumed, insulin can signal the body to store the energy from the food in the form of fat. Too much insulin results in too strong an impulse to eat, and makes your body too readily store food in the form of fat. To avoid carbohydrate addiction, you can minimize a high Glycemic Index (GI) value in choosing carbohydrate-rich foods as we explain in Chapter 12.

How many carbohydrates do you need?

The daily dietary reference intake (DRI) for carbohydrates is 45–65% of your daily Caloric need. Many dieticians recommend that about 50 percent of your daily Calories come from carbohydrates, this amounts to 284 grams of carbohydrates if you are on a 2,275 Calories diet. Like protein and fat, calculators on the Internet can give you a broad range for acceptable daily carbohydrate intake. You can calculate your recommended daily carbohydrate intake customized to your daily needs as follows: multiply your daily Caloric needs by the percent of Calories that you think you need from carbohydrates (e.g., 0.5 for 50%), then divide by 4 (number of Calories per gram of carb). Or simply, multiply your daily Calorie intake by 0.125 (which is 0.5 divided by 4). If you weigh 175 pounds (79 kilograms) and are on a 2,275 Calorie diet, you will need 2,275*0.125 = 284 grams of carbs per day.

Here is a short list to give you an idea of how many grams of carbs are in some foods: there are 26 grams of carb in a medium pear, 17 grams in 1 oz (28g) of dark chocolate, 53 grams in one cup (1/4L) of cooked white rice, 23 grams in one plain donut, and 5 grams in 24 almonds. There are many carbohydrate sources such as carrots, sweet potatoes, berries, persimmons, and apples that not only give your body and brain necessary fuel but also deliver essential vitamins and nutrients. The choice is yours, while keeping your Calories in check pick the one you like.

10.5 Fiber

Non-dietary fiber includes carbohydrates and other structural substances in plants that are indigestible to human enzymes. Fiber is made by plants to provide protection and structural support. Think about thick stems that help a plant stand upright, tough seed husks, and fruit skin that protect what is growing inside. You can find fiber in whole plant foods like whole grains, seeds, nuts, fruits, vegetables, and legumes. One of the most common types of fiber is cellulose, the main component in plant cell walls.

Dietary fiber is a carbohydrate, specifically a polysaccharide, which is incompletely absorbed in humans and in some animals. Like all carbohydrates, when it is metabolized, it can produce four Calories of energy per gram but, in most circumstances, it accounts for less than that because of its limited absorption and digestibility. The two subcategories are insoluble and soluble fiber.

Insoluble dietary fiber consists mainly of cellulose, a large carbohydrate polymer that is indigestible by humans, because humans do not have the required enzymes to break it down. Furthermore, the human digestive system does not harbor enough of the types of microbes that can do so.

Soluble dietary fiber comprises the following: a variety of oligosaccharides, waxes, esters, resistant starches, and other carbohydrates that dissolve or gelatinize in water. Many of these soluble fibers can be fermented or partially fermented by microbes in the human digestive system to produce short-chain fatty acids which are absorbed and therefore introduce some caloric content.

Beans, fruits especially plums, prunes, and figs, and vegetables are good sources of dietary fiber. Fiber is important to digestive health and is thought to reduce the risk of colon cancer. For mechanical reasons, fiber can help in alleviating both constipation and diarrhea. Fiber provides bulk to the intestinal contents, and insoluble fiber especially stimulates peristalsis—the rhythmic muscular contractions of the intestines which move digesta along the digestive tract. Some soluble fibers produce a solution of high viscosity that is essentially a gel, which slows the movement of food through the intestines. Additionally, fiber may help lessen insulin spikes and reduce the risk of type 2 diabetes.

How much fiber do you need?

Some research literature says people should be eating a minimum of 25g - 30g of fiber per day. This is how approximately 30g of fiber look like: half large avocado (4.5g fiber) + a cup (1/4L) of cooked lentils (4g fiber) + two carrots (6g fiber) + an apple with the skin on (4g fiber) + 2 cups kale boiled (5g fiber) + 3 oz of shiitake mushrooms (1.8 grams) + 6 oz raw broccoli (4.7g fiber). You may include your daily fiber need along with your overall daily recommended carbohydrate.

Chapter 11: What do You Eat? Quality over Quantity

A question many people ask us is "What do you eat?". In answer, we mostly cook our own food, so we know what's in it. We select our basic ingredients from correct foods, when possible. As we define it, correct foods include all kinds of foods but the correct version of them, as we will explain in the next chapter.

It is a lot healthier, a lot more fun, and a lot less expensive to cook your own food instead of packaged or restaurant foods. If you are eating the correct food made by you, then you may find you enjoy your food so much more, and that food prepared by outsiders holds little appeal. Also, the smell of roasted almonds and walnuts, and the aroma of chicken soup, pot roast, stews and other nice foods is very pleasant. Appendix C shows some of our favorite meals.

Spend your money on daily quality food, rather than splurging on drinking or eating out. Eating out or ordering in should not be a highly desired activity for finding enjoyment of regular food, or restaurant food for that matter. Home food should be what you like, and so good and good for you that there is no need to eat outside food regularly. In time, sugary-starchy-salty restaurant food becomes distasteful by comparison to your own real food. You should eat the correct foods you enjoy every day. However, once you reach your ideal weight, you can, on occasions, eat not-so-correct foods. Occasionally, we do eat not-so-correct foods, such as French bread, bagel, avocado-toast, turkey-avocado sandwich, egg salad sandwich, pizza, or even pancakes. Having bread occasionally makes it taste even more delicious than if we had it every day. Anticipation is half the joy! Better yet, having pancakes with lots of syrup might be an occasional guilty pleasure, but since we eat healthy food at home, we find we desire such things less and less.

Enjoy daily life rather than suffering today for a later future payoff. For example, if you like chocolate covered strawberries, why not eat them every morning, they are both tasty and nutritious, fun to make, and fun to eat. We cannot tell you how many times people have said: "But they are just for Christmas or Valentine's Day". Yet home prepared chocolate strawberries are not terribly expensive nor hard to make. And many people spend far more on drinking to mask stress. Why not have less stress and more happiness by doing what you want? Go ahead, make your day. Have chocolate covered strawberries whenever you want, especially when strawberries are in season. So yes, you can eat lots of fun things that are healthy as well. We will talk about how in the next chapter.

Most people in the developed world eat more than they should and too much of what they do not need, which can lead to a variety of health issues. Unfortunately, modern humans eat things that are not good for them and trap themselves in a fat corner. Then they find some quick-fix diet to fix it such as the variety of low-carb diets, which push them further down the fat corner creating a vicious circle. "Burn a little, save a lot" and fail at the end. So, they continue to eat the bad stuff that makes them fat and causes various health issues. The real fix to stay out of the fat corner, or better yet not to get into to begin with, is to maintain your Calories within your ideal weight, and equally important to focus on improving quality over quantity by choosing the correct food.

So, let's get to it!!

Chapter 12: How to Choose the Correct Food

With all the afore-mentioned potential nutritional pitfalls, what on earth can you eat? You could eat wild caught fish and seaweed all day every day, day after day but perhaps you prefer more variety. Variety is a source of pleasure that gives flavor to life, and literally more so when speaking of food. Sour, sweet, bitter, pungent, all must be tasted. The eye is pleased with the beautiful varieties of nature.

As we see it, just like you would choose cleaner brands of gasoline for your car to minimize engine deposits, increase vehicle performance, and improve fuel economy, the correct food provides the premium food fuel for your body's metabolic engine. So, you get "more bang for the buck", and less fat for the belly by using premium food fuel to create optimal ATP energy for your body to function at its best.

As you read this chapter, it may come as a surprise to you that some common foods are not the correct foods. Some of these are grains (particularly whole wheat), beans, legumes, nuts, fruits including tomatoes, some meat (including beef, fish, and chicken), dairy products, eggs, potatoes, eggplant, and peppers just to name a few.

The best correct foods contribute to minimizing fat savers and maximizing fat burners as we discussed in Chapter 7. As such, they should satisfy at least four criteria by having no: antinutrients such as lectins, toxins such as pesticides, unnatural substances such as artificial food additives, or antibiotics. They should also not be highly processed. Therefore, the best correct foods should have the following high standards:

- Fruits, vegetables, and nuts should be 100% organic.

- Fish and shellfish should be wild caught.

- Poultry should be pasture-raised (not just free-range) that consume some feed and lots of grass, bugs, worms, and anything else they can find in the dirt, and should usually be let out of the barns early in the morning and called back in before nightfall. In contrast to pastured-raised poultry, free-range animals may have more space than their caged and cage-free peers, but don't get outdoors as much as you may think. Some free-range chickens seldom get to see the light of day, and many eat corn, gluten, grain, or soy-based feed.

- Beef, milk, and dairy should be from grass-fed, grass-finished cattle that ate nothing but grass, not from cattle that are grass-fed and not grass-finished meaning they may only have had grass some time in their lifetime.

- Eggs should be from pasture-raised chickens.

These requirements for the best correct food are ideal but perhaps seemingly limiting your choices. You should work with what is available, and so choose the best correct food you can from available resources.

Below we will explain why some common foods are not the correct foods, and we will propose ways to choose the best correct foods you can so you can have a healthy version of the food you like. These are foods such as fruits and vegetables, meat and meat products, oil and fat, carbs, "nuts" and seeds, and food-for-thoughts.

Remember, you rebuild 1 to 2 percent of your muscle each day, meaning that you almost completely rebuild yourself every two to three months, and what you eat has a lot to do with how successfully your body is regenerated. So, you may wish to think carefully about what food you eat. Choose the correct food, so you keep rebuilding a healthier and a more energetic you.

12.1 Deciphering food labels

You might think food labels may help you in choosing the correct food. But here is the newsflash! Unfortunately, the food labeling may mislead you. Most of these labels are so convoluted that you may need a codebreaker to decode them! But, for simplicity, at least stay away from all products with the following food labels:

- "Gluten-free" generally means more sugar and lectins than gluten-containing products. Or the food may never have contained gluten in the first place such as fruits and vegetables. Don't pay extra for "gluten-free".

- "Grass-fed" means cattle may have had grass some time in their lifetime, but not necessarily all the time. Look for a grass-fed, grass-finished label instead, meaning cattle ate nothing but grass.

- "All natural" often means nothing and is not specifically defined, it may mean asbestos, arsenic, snake venom, a thunderstorm, and who knows what else.

- "All vegetarian feed" may mean lectins and genetically modified organisms (GMOs).

- "Free-range" may mean the chicken is fed grains, gluten, corn, and soy; and most chicken may not see the light of day albeit they are "allowed" to.

- "All organic ingredients" does not necessarily mean healthy. For example, organically raised GMO crops can be labeled organic too.

- "No artificial ingredients" may not be a guarantee of safety since non-artificial ingredients may contain questionable levels of non-artificial ingredients like natural chemicals such as monosodium glutamate (MSG), salt, or even arsenic, lead, and mercury.

- "No cholesterol", "No trans-fat", and "Partially hydrogenated" may mean bad omega 6. Or the food never contained cholesterol in the first place. For example, "no-cholesterol almond butter". Cholesterol is only found in animal products.

- "Sugar free", means artificial sweeteners.

- "Vegetable oil" may be high in lectins and/or LDL cholesterol.

12.2 Highly processed foods have no place in correct foods

In recent years, "processed food" has become synonymous with "unhealthy food". But make no mistake, not all processed foods are highly processed. Most people think all processed foods are created equally bad for you. Knowing the difference between healthy and harmful processing will help you shop smart and make the most informed choices when it comes to the correct foods.

There are big differences between processed foods and highly processed foods. Foods can go through various levels of processing. Any food that is processed is usually frozen, canned, dried, baked, or pasteurized. Yogurt is a processed food, vegetables that may only be cleaned, cut, and portioned before being sold in bags are processed food. Food cooked by you is also processed food. Unless you drink milk straight from a cow, eat shrimp right out of the ocean, or bite on an apple on the tree, most foods you eat are processed foods.

The most highly processed foods, however, are processed in an industrial process that is impossible for you to do domestically in your kitchen. Processing food to that degree strips out most of the protein and fiber along with the flavor. To put the flavor back they add extra sugar, salt, and fat. Watch out for the amount of that sugar, salt, and fat. With highly processed foods you get almost twice the daily recommended amount of sodium and sugar and a lot less protein and fiber than you need although it is cheaper.

Examples of highly processed foods comprise the following: frozen pizza, most frozen meals, chicken nuggets, French fries, soda, margarine, junk foods, and many breakfast cereals just to name a few.

Preservatives are also added to increase food's shelf life. It can be easy to overlook these additives in the list of ingredients. Watch out for terms such as dextrose, maltose, trans-fats, and hydrogenated oil.

To decide what food is highly processed, you can watch for additives and preservatives, or you can simply ask yourself, "could I recreate this myself at home or would I need a lab and a half dozen chemicals to do it?". We suggest an even better way: try to prepare your own meals from the basic ingredients chosen from the correct foods. In that way, since you don't eat them, you need not worry about the additives and preservatives on the food labels in pre-prepared foods, or what is in restaurant food for that matter.

12.3 How do we choose the correct fruits and vegetables?

Plants are smart traders. They give food to animals in exchange for their seeds and pollen taking a ride with and being spread around by the animals. They do not let the predators feed on them unless their seed husk is mature and ready for delivery by the predators. So, they use lectins as an anti-predator shield until they are ready to make the exchange.

Fruits come in a glorious rainbow of colors. Yellow, red, and orange fruits are not just pretty colors, they are communication signals from the fruit of peaceful surrender to the predators. The colors signal that the fruits are ripe and ready to feed the predators. Ripe fruit means the mature seed husk is hard and has its best chance of getting a ride through the predators' digestive tract unchanged and has a chance to survive and spread its seed. The percentage of lost seed is the price for the ride.

Thanks to the fruit industry, fruits may look ripe but may be artificially ripened. Fruit may be picked slightly unripe, transported, stored, and then exposed to ethylene gas on arrival at its destination. The ethylene gas exposure changes the color to make the fruit appear ripe and ready to eat. But induced colors are not the signals of peaceful surrender from the fruit to the predators, the fruit remains in counterattack mode. Not ready to get a ride for their seed husks with the predator to the broader world, their lectin's anti-predator shield remains active. Unlike naturally ripened fruit, the fruit never got the message from the parent plant to reduce lectin content. Because of human meddling in plants' affairs, no peaceful surrendering between the fruits and predators happens, the protective coating of the seed never fully matures, and the lectin content remains high. The high lectin count, when eating fruit picked too early, may be bad for your health.

How do you check whether the lectin anti-predator shield is active? Maybe take a Star Trek lectin tricorder to the grocery store with you. Maybe in the future, but until then you do not need to go to that length. Just choose fruits in season that are ripened naturally and not artificially ripened for year-round availability, select vegetables that are crisp and colorful, and preferably buy locally grown in season fruits and vegetables.

Correct fruits and vegetables comprise the following:

- 100% organic fruits: apple, apricots, avocados, berries, breadfruit, cherries, citrus fruits, coconuts, dates, figs, grapes, jackfruit, kiwis, nectarines, olives, peaches, pears, plums fresh or dried, pomegranates, and the like.

- 100% organic vegetables: artichokes, arugula, asparagus, baby greens, bamboo shoots, beets, Bok choy, broccoli, brussels sprouts, cabbages, carrots, cauliflower, celery, chicory, chives, collards, daikon radish, dandelion green, endive, escarole, fennel, garlic, ginger, hearts of palm, herbs (all kinds), kale, kimchi, kohlrabi, leeks, lemongrass, lettuces, mesclun, micro greens, mushrooms, lentils and red and white beans (properly pressure cooked), mustard green, okra, onions, purslane, radishes, raw sauerkraut, rhubarb, sea vegetables, seaweed, shallots, spinach, Swiss chard, water chestnuts, watercress, and the like.

In addition, you can choose from the following resistance starches year-round:

- Fruits: baobab fruit, green bananas, green mango, green papaya, green plantains, persimmon, and the like.
- Root vegetables: cassava, celery roots, glucomannan, jicama, parsnips, rutabaga, taro root, turnip, yam, yucca, and the like.

Avoid the following fruits and vegetables, unless you remove the seeds and skin from them and/or ferment them, since they are generally full of bad lectins.

- Fruits mistaken for vegetables: cantaloupe, cashews, chayote squash, cucumber, cucuzza squash, eggplant, gourd, luffa, pepper, pumpkin, summer squash, tomato, watermelon, zucchini, winter squash, and the like.
- Vegetables: corn and corn products, edamame, green beans, legumes (unless properly pressure cooked), pea protein, peas, soy products, soy, sprouts, and tofu.

12.4 How should we choose the correct meat and meat products?

If you eat meat, eat the correct meat. Eat meat without lectins. Wait a minute, cows are not plants. How do cows get lectins? Aren't cows supposed to eat grass? Yes, but thanks again to human interference they may not. The meat industry generally feeds cows with corn and soybeans full of lectins and who knows what else to add weight quickly and "make the weight requirement". Not only do cattle fed corn and soy gain weight faster but their meat also contains more fat marbling along with a more consistent taste. The same corn and grain in highly processed foods bulk you up as well, what goes around comes around your waist. In contrast, meat from grass-fed and grass-finished beef generally contains fewer Calories and less fat.

But corn and soybeans are not a cow's preferred way of eating.   During   the   evolutionary   process,   cattle discovered that if they can eat what others cannot, they can survive better.   So, they altered their method of digestion and passed it on to their offspring. Accordingly, cows can digest fibrous plant materials that humans, and most   animals   cannot.   Through   this   evolutionary process, cattle evolved with the mechanisms to eat and digest grass. Cows generally do not preferentially eat corn and soybeans force-fed to them by humans.

Because it is not natural for cows to eat large quantities of corn and soybeans, cows raised on it are more likely to suffer from these diets. Cows can develop heartburn from soybeans and corn just as you do. Since both corn and soy are full of lectins incompatible with cows' digestive system, they cause the cows to develop such severe stomach acid heartburn causing pain and swelling that they stop eating. Guess what some farmers do to force-feed them more. You guessed right, they feed the cows antacid in the form of calcium-carbonate, the active ingredient in many antacid tablets. Holy smokes! What have these cows done to humans to deserve such anti-cow treatment.

Our ancestors instinctively developed a host of ways to deal with anti-nutrients such as lectins. Unfortunately, many modern humans have not learned from their ancestors, and some may even think food comes from the Internet. Instead, many eat things that is not good for them and that can cause pain, heartburn, or discomfort. And to continue eating them, they find a quick fix remedy in antacids. But the remedy may be worse than the symptom because it may dramatically shift the balance of their microbiome toward bad bacteria, so they may keep craving those bad foods. They may not only continue eating foods that are bad for them, but they may also feed them to the farm animals they raise.

Even fish and poultry cannot escape the trend. Some farmers do similar things to the chickens and fish on their farms too. Some fish farmers have replaced traditional marine ingredients in fish feed with other ingredients such as corn and beans full of lectins. Also, farm-raised fish are generally fed with food full of omega-6 fatty acids which may cause an excessively high ratio of omega-6 to omega-3 fatty acids resulting in inflammation in the body of those who eat them. They may also add antibiotics to fish and chicken too, which may adversely affect the balance of your microbiome if you eat them. While there may be no evidence yet that antibiotics being consumed from animal food products cause harm to humans, they may increase resistance to targeted antibiotics when needed for treatment of infections in humans. We try to minimize antibiotics in our food anyway.

Wild caught fish, grass-fed and grass-finished cattle, and pasture-raised poultry and dairy are believed to be healthier albeit much more expensive. Cheaper feed may make the meat cheaper but may also make the animals, and whoever eats the animals, fatter. We want you to outsmart the food industry. Know your body and feed it with the correct food based both on your own knowledge and common sense. You can eat less but of higher quality, and thereby enjoy more with fewer Calories. If you choose the correct food, the increased volume may cause the food industry to make healthy food more accessible and less expensive.

Correct meat, dairy products, poultry, fish, and shellfish comprise the following:

- Grass-fed, grass-finished meat (minimize intake): beef, bison, boar, elk, lamb, pork, prosciutto, venison, wild game, and the like.

- Grass-fed, grass-finished dairy products (in moderation): buffalo butter, buffalo mozzarella butter, caw butter (A-2/France, Italy, or Switzerland), French/Italian butter, ghee, goat butter; A-2 blue cheese, caw ricotta (A-2/Italy), French/Italian cheese, goat cheese, Parmesan-Reggiano cheese, sheep cheese, Switzerland cheese; caw milk (A-2/France, Italy, or Switzerland), goat milk; caw yogurt (A-2), coconut yogurt, plain goat yogurt, plain sheep yogurt; goat and sheep kefir; organic cream cheese, organic heavy cream, organic sour cream; whey protein powder, and the like.

- Wild caught fish and shellfish: Alaskan salmon, anchovies, freshwater bass, Hawaiian fish, kipper, mahi-mahi, sardines, skipjack tuna, whitefish; calamari, clams, crab, lobster, mussels, oysters, scallops, shrimp, and the like.

- Pastured-raised poultry: chicken, dove, duck, goose, grouse, ostrich, pheasant, quail, turkey, wild game, pastured-raised eggs, and the like.

What about fake meats? We are a NO on that one. They generally contain huge amounts of lectins. If that is not enough, they may contain herbicides (e.g., glyphosate), which may be deadly disruptors to your health and life span. We would not be surprised if in the future you see commercials, saying: "If you have been eating fake meat, and been diagnosed with this disease or that disease, let this law firm help you". Also, if you eat fake meat because you think it has less fat than the real one, think again. Fake meat may have even more fat than real meat. The bottom line is that fake meat is a highly processed food, and, as you know, highly processed foods have no place in the correct foods. If you do not eat meat, eat lentils instead, not fake meat please. Eat the real thing.

12.5 How to choose the correct oil and fat?

As we mentioned in Chapter 10, unsaturated fat ("good-fat") has many health benefits unlike saturated fat ("not-so-good fat") and trans fats ('bad-fat") that may negatively impact health. Having reminded you of that: correct oil should be unsaturated, saturated fat such as those in meat and dairy listed above should be consumed in moderation, and trans fats should be eliminated.

Correct sources of oil comprise the following:

• Algae oil, flaxseed oil, MCT oil, macadamia oil, sesame oil, perilla oil, hempseed oil, red palm oil, walnut oil, extra virgin olive oil, avocado oil, and the like.

Incorrect sources of oil comprise the following:

• Vegetable (e.g., corn and soy), peanut, canola, grape seed, cottonseed, sunflower, safflower, and the like. Note: although many of these oils are also considered unsaturated, they may have a high quantity of anti-nutrients such as lectins.

12.6 How about the correct carbs?

Having carbohydrates is not a bad thing. Rather it is having the wrong carbohydrates such as simple sugars, corn syrup, high fructose corn syrup, and excessive consumption of carbohydrates that is not so good. The correct carbs are good carbs which comprise most complex carbohydrates, and particularly those that are nutrient-rich with moderate and preferably low glycemic Index (GI).

GI is a relative ranking of carbohydrates in foods according to how they affect blood glucose levels. Carbohydrates with a low GI value (e.g., 55 or less) are usually more slowly digested, absorbed, and metabolized, and generally cause a lower and slower rise in blood glucose and therefore slower rise in insulin levels.

But this brings us to a broader point. The GI is still just a list of numbers. How a food specifically affects someone's unique makeup and blood sugar varies by individual. You can find GI values of most foods on the Internet. As for us, with the exception of beets that have moderate GI (e.g., 55-69), we mostly eat carbohydrates with low GI values.

In addition to the fruits, vegetables, dairy products, and oil listed above, correct carbohydrates with acceptable GI values comprise the following:

- Flours: almond, cassava, coconut, grape seed, green banana, hazelnut, sesame, sweet potato, tiger nut, and the like.

- Dark chocolate.

- Nuts and seeds: see the next section.

Minimize high GI value (e.g., 70-100) carbohydrate-rich foods, since they may cause carbohydrate addiction, if you don't. As we mentioned in Chapter 10, carbohydrate-rich foods increase insulin level, and an increase in insulin level increases craving, and an increase in craving can cause carbohydrate addiction.

Carbohydrate-rich foods may comprise the following:

- Starches/flour: arrowroot flour, bagels, breakfast cereals, chestnut flour, cornstarch, crackers, pasta, popcorn, potato chips, potatoes, pretzels, rice flour, rice, tortillas, wheat breads, wheat flour, whole grain flour, whole wheat flour spelt, and the like.

- Sweets: cakes, cookies, corn syrup, Danishes, donuts, ice cream, pastry, pie, sugar-sweetened beverages, table sugar, and the like.

- All fruit juices, and highly processed foods, because they are high in sugar that can increase your insulin level. Next time somebody says orange juice is healthy, think about this: an 8 fl. oz (237mL) glass of orange juice has 1.6 tablespoons (20g) of sugar equal to 1.16 tablespoons (24.3g) of honey.

- Most restaurant foods.

- Most alcoholic beverages.

To further minimize high GI value (e.g., 70-100) carbohydrate-rich foods in your diet, you can also replace your bread-based foods with protein-based foods and minimize sugar and alcohol. For a non-diabetic, you may not necessarily need to have a sugar-free diet but reducing the amount of sugar you consume is probably a wise decision. In addition, carbohydrate act-a-likes such as alcoholic beverages, monosodium glutamate and sugar substitutes may trigger intense or recurring carbohydrate cravings and associated weight gain. So, if you would like to fit in your skinny clothes again, as in our *Lowellie*™ *Way*, start by eliminating "bread" and reducing starches/flour from your daily diet, at least for the first few months. Subsequently, you can replace bread, for example, with tortillas made with cassava and coconut flour, or almond flour (with blanched almonds), and the like. Or, if you really miss your good old "bread", you can eat it occasionally like we do.

Bear in mind, if you are eating a lot more Calories per day than you are burning, then your liver will convert excess Calories into fat, no matter whether it is from high GI value carbohydrates (like simple sugar), or low GI value carbohydrates (like fruits). All good reasons to keep your Calories in check.

Also beware that sugar can operate covertly! Look for the following items on the ingredients label, they are all forms of sugar: corn syrup, high fructose corn syrup, fructose, molasses, honey, fruit juice concentrate, and white, brown, raw or cane sugar. Some people tell us: "I do not eat sugar, I only eat honey", *well*, honey is sugar too. Look for the quantity of sugar listed on the "Nutrition Facts" panel of the foods you buy. It will be listed in grams. Remember, no matter what the source is, be it the natural fructose in strawberries or the added sweetness of corn syrup, it all winds up in the same place on the nutrition facts label. If a product only lists fresh or dried fruit in the ingredients list, you know that the sugar is derived from these sources. However, if cane sugar and corn syrup are listed in addition to the strawberries, you know that sugars have been added. By the way, yogurt has sugar too, no need to add honey or fruit to it.

Fruits are sneaky too, the fructose half of sugar in fruits can cause you to become resistant to your main appetite suppression hormones (insulin and leptin). When this happens, your appetite is not shut down when it should be, and you just keep eating. Therefore, you can eat a lot of fruit before you know you have had enough, and your weight may accelerate out of control.

Finally, remember grains have bad lectins. As we explained in the previous chapters, bad lectins are fat savers. They bind to cell membranes and can cause inflammation and thus promote storing excess fat in the fat cells. If you absolutely cannot give up grains, no matter how hard you try, always choose refined "white" grains over whole grains. Do not go for brown rice, go for white rice such as white Basmati rice. Do not eat whole wheat bread, find the healthiest version of white bread if you can. Even though lots of people think brown rice is better for them than white rice, people whose cultures have always eaten rice usually stripped the hull from brown rice before they ate it. Why? Because they know that the hull is where all the harmful lectins live.

12.7 How to choose the correct nuts and seeds

To start with, some nuts and seeds contain five different anti-nutrients: Oxalic acid, Phytic acid, Lectins, Tannins, and Trypsin Inhibitors. Each of these naturally occurring compounds deplete a wide array of essential micronutrients that your body needs to obtain and

Nut Anti-Nutrient	Micronutrients Depleted by the Nut Anti-Nutrient
Lectins	Most Vitamins and Minerals
Tannins	Iron, Calcium, Magnesium, Zinc, Vitamins B1 and B9
Oxalic Acid	Iron, Calcium, Magnesium
Trypsin Inhibitors	Vitamins A, D, E, K, and amino acids
Phytic Acid	Iron, Calcium, Magnesium, Copper, Chromium, Manganese, Zinc, Vitamins B3 and D

achieve optimal health. To put that into perspective, that is more than any other single food in the world! This is illustrated in the following table.

Nonetheless, nuts are full of beneficial nutrition, and we should eat them because we like them. But some nuts, like almonds, are high in anti-nutrients and you should have them with a "grain of salt", literally that is. To get the correct version of almonds, soak them in warm water and salt and rinse them after soaking. By soaking you can remove or eliminate most of the anti-nutrients which are mostly on their skin. You can also or alternatively blanch the almonds to remove the skin. You can also roast them after soaking if you like. We like roasted almonds.

Correct nuts and seeds comprise the following:

- Nuts: almonds blanched (without skins) or properly soaked, almond butter from blanched almonds, baruka nuts, Brazil nuts, chestnuts, coconut, macadamia nuts, pecans, nut butters, pine nuts, pistachios, and the like.
- Seeds: flax, hemp protein powder, hemp, poppy, psyllium, sesame, and the like.

Also, eliminate the following incorrect nuts and seeds since they have high lectins:

- Seeds: chia, pumpkin, and sunflower.
- Nuts: peanuts and cashews.

Peanuts and cashews are not technically nuts and have special properties of their own. Peanuts are legumes, not nuts, and are loaded with killer lectins. About 94% of people may carry a preformed antibody to the peanut's lectin, but peanut allergies can be life-threatening to some people. Cashews are beans that hang separately from the fruit. Because of its potent lectins, Amazonians take the Cashew's "nut" away and eat only the fruit. In some people, cashews and cashew nut butter have caused outbreaks of rashes after consuming. No wonder, cashews are in the same botanical family as poison ivy. Cashews have also been shown to cause inflammation in some people.

12.8 How to choose the correct grains and legumes

Our ancestors, unbeknownst to them, reduced or entirely removed anti-nutrients like lectins by soaking, fermentation, deseeding, peeling, and pressure cooking. Why shouldn't we? Pressure cooking is on a par with fermentation as the best way to reduce the lectins in grains. It turns out, pressure cooking may be the best way to cook your beans and grains!

Correct grains and legumes that you can pressure cook to remove anti-nutrients comprise the following:

- Grains: amaranth, quinoa, white rice, and the like.
- Legumes: beans, chickpeas, lentils, and the like.

Eliminate the following grains from your diet since lectins from gluten containing grains generally cannot be eliminated (i.e., pressure cooking would probably not work):

- Barley, brown rice, bulgur, oats, rye, wheat, and the like.

12.9 How do we choose the correct food-for-thoughts?

To maintain a healthy and happy lifestyle, Calories, correct food, and hormones all matter. There is no denying a fundamental law. A Calorie deficit should exist for your metabolism to dip into stored energy. You get there by keeping your Calories within the Calories of your ideal weight.

You eat the correct food and exercise to keep your metabolism day after day from adapting and slowing down, manage cravings, increase energy, and control appetite surges. But how do you keep the momentum going, what keeps you from slowing down in your quest to reach your ideal weight? That has everything to do with "happiness hormones": oxytocin, endorphins, serotonin, and dopamine. For simplicity, think of all the hormones in your body as musicians in a symphony orchestra of your metabolism that play together. And further, think of happiness hormones as a subset of these musicians that play the Allegro (cheerful music) inspired by the correct food-for-thoughts.

A balanced diet of the correct food and exercise can go a long way in keeping you happy. As we define it, correct food-for-thoughts is a combination of correct food and exercise, that more specifically activates the happiness hormones. Happiness hormones give you a head full of happy thoughts, bring you up out of your chair, get you skipping around the room, and change your feeling to one of complete energy. In the next few sections, we will discuss happiness hormones and how you can activate them by the correct food-for-thoughts.

The love maker

Oxytocin is a hormone and a neurotransmitter. Oxytocin often called the "love hormone" that can help promote trust, empathy, and bonding in relationships. Oxytocin levels generally increase with physical affection like kissing, cuddling, and sex. Oxytocin production can be stimulated by a variety of the correct food, especially ones containing vitamin D, vitamin C, magnesium, and dietary fats.

Most fruits and vegetables have vitamin C. We mostly choose the following correct fruits and vegetables: spinach, citrus fruits, berries, apples, pears, grapes, and avocado. There are many ways to increase your vitamin D. For example, sunshine produces vitamin D through a chemical reaction in your skin, or you can eat fatty fish, mushrooms, and eggs. Green leafy vegetables, nuts and seeds are a good source of magnesium. Eating a variety of fats, even saturated fat and cholesterol, helps with hormone production including oxytocin. As our major source of fat, we eat correct fats such as salmon, dark chocolate, almonds, walnuts, avocado, olive oil, and avocado oil. While excess cholesterol may not be good for us, our body needs it in the proper amounts. Cholesterol can be found in fatty fish such as salmon, seeds, or nuts.

Managing stress is a critical part of keeping hormones healthy. Oxytocin can be affected with stress. When you are stressed, your cortisol level goes up and your oxytocin level goes down. Exercise is a great way to keep stress down and oxytocin levels up. One of our favorite fun activities to increase oxytocin is to eat chocolate covered strawberries and dance tango under the sunlight.

The pleasure maker

Endorphins are hormones and neurotransmitters. In the brain they act as pain relievers and natural opiates without the same addiction risk. These chemical messengers are like opiate drugs such as morphine but are significantly stronger. Endorphins are associated with emotions and pain perception, and your brain produces them in response to fear or trauma to reduce the feeling of stress and increase pleasure.

Even the anticipation of an experience can increase endorphins, which may explain their role in the placebo effect. As pleasurable and safe as the effects of endorphins are on the brain, it is only natural to want to increase them. While a sustained release is not possible due to the quick assimilation of the chemical into the body, it is possible to incorporate small endorphin spikes throughout the day.

Humans increase endorphins daily by engaging in activities that feel good as the result of release of these pain-blocking neurotransmitters. Endorphin-releasing activities comprise, for example, exercise, eating, dancing, and laughter. Other activities that cause either pain or stress, and can increase endorphins comprise, for example, childbirth, light to moderate drinking, and exposure to ultraviolet light. Perhaps the best-known way to increase endorphins is exercise. The type of exercise is important. Moderately strenuous exercise raises endorphin levels more than gentle exercise. It is not only endorphins, however, that are responsible for the runner's high. Other brain chemicals, like serotonin and adrenaline, are likely involved.

Some activities associated with milder types of physical stress are believed to increase endorphins. Exercises that use controlled breathing, like yoga and tai chi, release endorphins and increase feelings of well-being and peace. Getting a massage or having acupuncture may have a similar effect on endorphin levels.

Eating capsaicin-containing foods like hot chili peppers can cause an endorphin release in response to the pain of eating them. Chocolate, sweet foods, and fatty foods can cause release of a powerful endorphin called beta-endorphin that can relieve pain. This is partially responsible for the feelings of well-being people experience after eating carbohydrates. This makes carbohydrates addictive. Make sure you do not "overdose" on endorphin by eating excessive cakes. Limit your carbs and laugh a little longer instead.

Laughter is another simple way to increase endorphin levels. The act of laughing may have many effects such as lifting mood, increasing immunity, and reducing the harmful effects of stress on the body. Regular laughter has been shown in studies to reduce the symptoms of depression.

Delightful you

Serotonin is a hormone and a neurotransmitter that helps to regulate many of your brain functions such as mood, sleep, appetite, digestion, learning ability, and memory. Serotonin is produced by long-term cardio exercise and may improve agreeable social interaction. Serotonin is not found in foods, but a precursor amino acid tryptophan is. Food high in protein, iron, riboflavin, and vitamin B-6 such as milk, yogurt, eggs, red meat, chicken, and salmon all tend to contain large amounts of tryptophan. While high-tryptophan foods will not boost serotonin on their own, there is one possible cheat to this system, carbs. Carbs cause the body to release more insulin, which promotes amino acid absorption and leaves tryptophan in the blood.

No mountain is too high

Dopamine is known as the "feel-good" hormone and is a hormone and a neurotransmitter that is an important part of your brain's reward system. Dopamine is a neurotransmitter that our brain produces to nudge us into doing things. Dopamine is a main reason why we can focus and achieve great things even if the payout is not immediate or obvious. Dopamine is associated with thought and pleasurable feelings and is released during pleasurable situations such as creating relationships or learning something new. This hormone causes you to seek out that pleasure feeling repeatedly.

You can increase dopamine to increase productivity. You increase dopamine in your system to help you stay focused, productive, and motivated. Aside from being the ultimate motivator, having a constant supply of dopamine in your system has a few other fringe benefits: helps you lose weight, makes you feel more alive, improves your memory, may stop self-destructive behavior including certain addictions, may counteract depression, let's you resist impulsive behavior, and may help you avoid Parkinson's disease.

You can boost your dopamine levels by increasing your Tyrosine. Tyrosine is a main amino acid building block of dopamine, so make sure that you have enough of this amino acid in you. Fortunately, it is easy enough to find Tyrosine. Here are some common foods that have loads of tyrosine: almonds, avocados, bananas, beef, chicken, chocolate, coffee, eggs, green tea, milk, and yogurt.

You can also add turmeric to your diet. Turmeric inhibits monoamine oxidase (MAO) enzymes preventing neurotransmitter depletion, and aids serotonin and dopamine production to restore healthy neurotransmitters. Turmeric may also create more neurotransmitter receptors by promoting neurogenesis. You can add turmeric to your food, coffee and other drinks or take it as a pill.

12.10 Shoot for the stars

To maintain a healthy lifestyle, it is good to maintain a healthy weight. For that, our message is simple. Eat the correct food in a correct amount and exercise regularly. This may create a fat burning state with premium food fuel in which your body is ready to burn the fat, instead of making and trapping it. In the fat burning environment your insulin and cortisol are low, and anti-nutrients are reduced or eliminated.

Ready to burn the fat now? What you must do is to breathe! Want to burn more? Breathe more!! Want to burn even more and eat less? Add extra protein. Want to keep it going? Activate happiness hormones and make a head full of happy thoughts. Finally, all roads lead to ATP, where you get the big bang for the buck, your ATP production goes through the roof. Why? because your mitochondria are happy too, not overworked, they have the capacity to generate whatever immediate energy you need for whatever activity you want. Got ideas? Dancing?

You may say a perfect fat burning state may not be possible, yes life is not about perfection, but rather minimizing risk while aiming high. So, we say "shoot for the stars and you might hit the streetlight". Or better yet, shoot for the stars, and you may hit your target weight! Either way you might hit a home run.

12.11 Use your common sense

You do the best you can with the information you have. Trust your common sense, not what "Experts" say. Any change in lifestyle should be over an extended time to allow adjustment time. Many have seen numerous diet fads throughout the ages that push bad food on you. Once upon a time, breakfast cereal and soda were considered health food but now they are mostly sugary, full of bad lectins, and not so good for you. Some in the food industry are trying to push fad diets, supplements, and fake meat on you, and sooner or later you may find these are not so good either.

To this end what makes sense to us is to eat what we like, but the correct version of it. We do not follow a strict lectin-free, fat-free, and sugar-free diet. We are mindful of antinutrients, saturated fat and sugar and try to minimize them. In a nutshell, we try to reduce the fat savers and increase the fat burners by having a balanced diet of the correct food within the calories of our ideal weight and exercise regularly.

Epilogue

Lose Weight and Keep Healthy and Energetic

We wrote this book because so many people want to copy our lifestyle. So, in this book we outlined some of the things related to diet that work for us. As always, consider your own situation and consult your own physician or nutritionist. For those who wish to copy our lifestyle, our basic concept is to use common sense rather than follow fads. The title of the book refers to the tendency of many dieting advertisements to add the phrase "... along with a balanced diet and exercise" to whatever product or service they are advertising. However, if you have a balanced diet of the correct food within the Calories of your ideal weight and exercise regularly, you may get the desired result anyway. Or maybe, you get an even better result without the need for fad diets and diet products.

We ignore silly diets and diet products since with our Lowellie™ Way to a healthy lifestyle you can get good results anyway. So, you can dance a little longer, laugh a little louder, hold hands a little tighter, kiss like your heart wants to thunder, and find the happiness that thrills you with wonder ☺.

Appendix A: Ideal Weight Chart

Male		Female	
Height	**Ideal Body Weight**	**Height**	**Ideal Body Weight**
4' 6" (137cm)	63-77 lbs. (29-35kg)	4' 6" (137cm)	63-77 lbs. (29-39kg)
4' 7" (140cm)	68-84 lbs. (31-38kg)	4' 7" (140cm)	68-83 lbs. (31-38kg)
4' 8" (142cm)	74-90 lbs. (34-41kg)	4' 8" (142cm)	72-88 lbs. (33-40kg)
4' 9" (145cm)	79-97 lbs. (36-44kg)	4' 9" (145cm)	77-94 lbs. (35-43kg)
4' 10" (147cm)	85-103 lbs. (39-47kg)	4' 10" (147cm)	81-99 lbs. (37-45kg)
4' 11" (150cm)	90-110 lbs. (41-50kg)	4' 11" (150cm)	86-105 lbs. (39-48kg)
5' 0" (152cm)	95-117 lbs. (43-53kg)	5' 0" (152cm)	90-110 lbs. (41-50kg)
5' 1" (155cm)	101-123 lbs. (46-56kg)	5' 1" (155cm)	95-116 lbs. (43-53kg)
5' 2" (157cm)	106-130 lbs. (48-59kg)	5' 2" (157cm)	99-121 lbs. (45-55kg)
5' 3" (160cm)	112-136 lbs. (51-62kg)	5' 3" (160cm)	104-127 lbs. (47-58kg)
5' 4" (162cm)	117-143 lbs. (53-65kg)	5' 4" (162cm)	108-132 lbs. (49-60kg)
5' 5" (165cm)	122-150 lbs. (55-68kg)	5' 5" (165cm)	113-138 lbs. (51-63kg)
5' 6" (168cm)	128-156 lbs. (58-71kg)	5' 6" (168cm)	117-143 lbs. (53-65kg)
5' 7" (170cm)	133-163 lbs. (60-74kg)	5' 7" (170cm)	122-149 lbs. (55-68kg)
5' 8" (173cm)	139-169 lbs. (63-77kg)	5' 8" (173cm)	126-154 lbs. (57-70kg)
5' 9" (175cm)	144-176 lbs. (65-80kg)	5' 9" (175cm)	131-160 lbs. (59-73kg)
5' 10" (178cm)	149-183 lbs. (68-83kg)	5' 10" (178cm)	135-165 lbs. (61-75kg)
5' 11" (180cm)	155-189 lbs. (70-86kg)	5' 11" (180cm)	140-171 lbs. (64-78kg)
6' 0" (183cm)	160-196 lbs. (73-89kg)	6' 0" (183cm)	144-176 lbs. (65-80kg)
6' 1" (185cm)	166-202 lbs. (75-92kg)	6' 1" (185cm)	149-182 lbs. (68-83kg)
6' 2" (188cm)	171-209 lbs. (78-95kg)	6' 2" (188cm)	153-187 lbs. (69-87kg)
6' 3" (191cm)	176-216 lbs. (80-98kg)	6' 3" (191cm)	158-193 lbs. (72-88kg)
6' 4" (193cm)	182-222 lbs. (83-101kg)	6' 4" (193cm)	162-198 lbs. (74-90kg)
6' 5" (196cm)	187-229 lbs. (85-104kg)	6' 5" (196cm)	167-204 lbs. (76-93kg)
6' 6" (198cm)	193-235 lbs. (88-107kg)	6' 6" (198cm)	171-209 lbs. (78-95kg)
6' 7" (201cm)	198-242 lbs. (90-110kg)	6' 7" (201cm)	176-215 lbs. (80-98kg)
6' 8" (203cm)	203-249 lbs. (92-113kg)	6' 8" (203cm)	180-220 lbs. (82-100kg)
6' 9" (206cm)	209-255 lbs. (95-116kg)	6' 9" (206cm)	185-226 lbs. (84-103kg)
6' 10" (208cm)	214-262 lbs. (97-119kg)	6' 10" (208cm)	189-231 lbs. (86-105kg)
6' 11" (211cm)	220-268 lbs. (100-122kg)	6' 11" (211cm)	194-237 lbs. (88-108kg)
7' 0" (213cm)	225-275 lbs. (102-125kg)	7' 0" (213cm)	198-242 lbs. (90-110kg)

The original ideal body weight chart was developed by MET Life, 1943.

Appendix B: Quick Calorie Chart (QCC)*

Food Category	Food Item	Food Amount	Cal** (kcal)	Fat (grams)	Carbs (grams)	Protein (grams)
Dairy	A2 yogurt	1 oz	20	1.2	1.5	1
Dairy	A2 light milk	8 fl oz	106	3	12	7.5
Eggs	Egg white	1 large	17	0	0	4
Eggs	Whole eggs	1 large	78	5	0.6	6
Fruit	Apple - 3" diameter	1 medium	95	0.3	25	0.5
Fruit	Avocado 1/2	medium	125	12	8	2.5
Fruit	Blue berries	1	1	0	0.2	0
Fruit	Cherries - sweet	1	4	0	1.1	0.1
Fruit	Persimmon - Fuyu 2.5"	1	118	0.3	31	1
Grain (cooked)	Lentil	1 cup	230	0.8	40	18
Grain (cooked)	Rice - white Basmati	1 cup	205	0.4	45	4.3
Meat	NY strip steak	1 oz	60	3	0	8
Meat	Ham - lean deli sliced	1 oz	31	0.8	0.8	5
Meat - poultry	Chicken breast - skinless	1 oz	31	35	0	6.5
Meat - poultry	Turkey breast	1 oz	30	0.25	0	6
Meat - seafood	Cod - boneless	1 oz	49	2.5	1.9	4.4
Meat - seafood	Salmon - wild Atlantic	1 oz	40	1.8	0	6
Meat - seafood	Shrimp - steamed	1 large	12	0	0	3
Meat - seafood	Smoked salmon - lox	1 oz	55	7	0	5.5
Nuts - tree nuts	Almonds	1	7	0.6	0.2	0.3
Nuts - tree nuts	Pistachios	1	4	0.3	0.2	0.1
Oil - fruit oil	Avocado oil	1 tbsp	124	14	0	0

* The nutritional facts listed in the QCC are based on nutrition facts labels approved by the USA Food and Drug Administration (FDA) only within a margin of error of up to about 20 percent. But they are still useful to give you a general sense of your nutrition intake per day and to compare options to see which is better.

** The Calories in the QCC are kilocalories (symbol: Cal). Kilocalories are approximately the amount of energy needed to raise the temperature of one kilogram of water by one degree Celsius. For example, it takes the energy in 0.1-gram olive oil to heat a kilogram of water one degree Celsius. Kilocalories (kcal) may also be known as food calories, large calories, kilogram calories, dietary calories, nutritionist's calories, nutritional calories. Kilocalories equal 1000 small calories (symbol: cal).

Appendix C: Some of Our Favorite Meals

Breakfast

Smoked Salmon and egg white

Ingredients per serving

Food Item	Amount	Nutrition Facts			
		Calories (kcal)	Fat (grams)	Carb (grams)	Protein (grams)
Smoked Salmon (lux)	4 oz	220	28	0	22
Egg white	6	102	0	0	24
Avocado oil	1/2 tbsp	65	7	0	0
Chocolate - dark	1 oz	150	9	17	1.4
		537	44	17	47

Method ☺

1. Brush a medium non-stick frying pan with the 1/2 tbsp of the avocado oil.
2. Pour the egg white into the pan, cook for 5 minutes over medium heat or until surface is nearly firm.
3. Place the smoked salmon on the egg white.
4. Enjoy the chocolate on the side.

Breakfast

Egg white omelet with spinach and ham

Ingredients per serving

Food Item	Amount	Nutrition Facts			
		Calories (kcal)	Fat (grams)	Carb (grams)	Protein (grams)
Avocado oil	1 tbsp	124	14	0	0
Egg white	6 large	102	0	0	24
Ham - lean deli sliced	4 oz	124	3.2	3	20
Spinach	6 oz	42	0.3	3	2.4
Almond butter cookie	1	135	10	4	4
Dark chocolate-covered strawberry	1 large	60	4	6	0.1
		587	32	16	58

Method

1. Brush a medium non-stick frying pan with 1/2 tbsp of the avocado oil.
2. Pour the egg white into the pan.
3. Place the spinach on top of the egg white and cover the pan with a lid.
4. Place the pan over medium heat, cook for 5 minutes or until spinach is wilted.
5. Meanwhile, brush another medium non-stick frying pan with the other 1/2 tbsp of the avocado oil.
6. Chop the ham and sauté for 5 minutes in the pan.
7. Place the ham over half the egg white and spinach, then fold over the other side to enclose the filling.
8. Optional spices et al.: 1/2 tsp turmeric, 1/2 tsp black pepper, 1 pinch of salt, and/or 1 tbsp grounded organic flax seeds.
9. Enjoy the strawberries and cookies on the side.

Lunch or dinner

Wild Atlantic Salmon

Ingredients per serving

Food Item	Amount	Calories (kcal)	Fat (grams)	Carb (grams)	Protein (grams)
Skinless wild Atlantic salmon	6 oz	240	10.8	0	36
Baby spinach	3 oz	21	0.3	3	2.4
Beets - cooked and sliced	6 oz	72	0.3	16.2	2.8
Balsamic vinegar - white	1 tbsp	10	0	3	0
Olive oil	1 tbsp	130	14	0	0
		473	**25**	**22**	**41**

Method ☺

1. Bring the salmon to room temperature 10 minutes before cooking. Warm a large non-stick frying pan with the ½ tbsp of the oil over medium-low heat. Season the fish with salt to taste. Raise the heat to medium-high. Place the salmon, in the pan. Cook until golden brown on 1 side, about 5 minutes. Turn the fish over with a spatula and cook until it feels firm to the touch and the skin is crisp if desired, about 4 minutes more.
2. In a large mixing bowl add the baby spinach, beets, avocado, vinegar, and the remaining 1/2 tbsp of olive oil. Toss lightly and transfer to a salad serving bowl. Top it with the salmon or serve it separately.
3. Enjoy the yogurt on the side.

Lunch or dinner

Turkey Avocado Plate with Stuffed Bella Mushrooms
Turkey Avocado Plate

Ingredients per serving

Food Item	Amount	Nutrition Facts			
		Calories (kcal)	Fat (grams)	Carb (grams)	Protein (grams)
Turkey breast - oven browned, sliced	7 oz	210	1.75	0	42
Avocado - medium, sliced	1/2	125	12	8	2.5
Stuffed Bella mushrooms *	2	190	19.3	2.4	1.2
Apple	1	95	0.3	25	1.2
		620	**33**	**35**	**47**

Method 😊

1. Place the turkey slices on a plate.
2. Place the avocado slices on the turkey.
3. Place the stuffed mushrooms on the turkey plate.

*Stuffed Bella Mushrooms**

Ingredients per serving

Food Item	Amount	Nutrition Facts			
		Calories (kcal)	Fat (grams)	Carb (grams)	Protein (grams)
Baby bella mushroom - medium	1	4	0.06	0.6	0.6
Olive oil	1/2 tbsp	65	7	0	0
Walnuts	2 halves	26	2.6	1.2	0.6
		95	**10**	**2**	**1**

Method 😊

1. Wipe 2 baby bella mushrooms off with a damp paper towel to clean. Carefully pop the stems out of the caps. You can use the mushroom caps raw or toss them with a little olive oil until tender.
2. Add 2 walnuts haves to each mushroom cap.
3. Sprinkle1/2 tbsp olive oil on the walnut halves on each mushroom cap.

Lunch or dinner

Chef Salad

Ingredients per serving

Food Item	Amount	Nutrition Facts			
		Calories (kcal)	Fat (grams)	Carb (grams)	Protein (grams)
Butterhead lettuce - bite-size pieces	1 head	21	0.4	3.6	2.2
Chicken breast - boneless skinless	6 oz	186	210	0	39
Avocado - medium, bite-size pieces	1/2	125	12	8	2.5
Blue cheese - crumbled	1 oz	100	8	0.7	6
Whole egg - hard boiled, chopped	1	78	5	0.6	6
Olive oil	1 tbsp	130	14	0	0
Balsamic vinegar - white	1 tbsp	10	0	3	0
		650	**249**	**16**	**56**

Method 😊

1. Broil the chicken with your favorite recipe and cut it in bite-size pieces.
2. In a large mixing bowl add the lettuce, chicken breast, avocado, egg, and blue cheese. Add olive oil, and vinegar.
3. Toss lightly and transfer to a salad serving bowl.

Lunch or dinner

Chicken Soup
(Only occasionally)

Ingredients per serving

Food Item	Amount	Nutrition Facts			
		Calories (kcal)	Fat (grams)	Carb (grams)	Protein (grams)
Chicken breast - boneless skinless	7 oz	217	245	0	45.5
Avocado - medium, bite-size pieces	1/2	125	12	8	2.5
White Basmati rice - cooked	2/3 cup	153	0.3	0	3.2
Picante Sauce	4 tbsp	20	0	4	0
A2 yogurt	6 oz	120	7.2	9	6
Celery	3 stocks	21	0	6	0
		656	**265**	**27**	**57**

Method ☺

1. Cook the rice with your favorite recipe.
2. Boil the chicken breast with your favorite recipe. Separate the chicken and the cooking water. Shred the chicken.
3. Place the shredded chicken, rice, and avocado in a soup bowl, add the picante sauce on the top. Add about 1 cup of the cooking water to the soup bowl.
4. Enjoy the celery and the yogurt on the side.

About The Authors

Lowell and Elahe live roughly as outlined above, and friends and neighbors frequently marvel at their love for each other as they hug and kiss and dance Argentine Tango. They are highly educated and experienced engineers, philosophers, and intellectual property professionals. Combined they have a Doctor of Philosophy degree, 3 Master of Science degrees, and 2 Bachelor of Science degrees.